CW00557643

 The**inspirational**series™
Overcoming adversity and thriving

Unbroken
Learning to Live Beyond Diagnosis
BY ALEXIS QUINN

We are proud to introduce The**inspirational**series™. Part of the Trigger family of innovative mental health books, The**inspirational**series™ tells the stories of the people who have battled and beaten mental health issues. For more information visit: www.triggerpublishing.com

THE AUTHOR

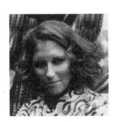 Alexis Quinn, from Morecombe Cove, now resident of Lagos, is a gifted academic, teacher, and former professional athlete. A passionate educator, she has worked within the education system for over a decade. After being wrongly diagnosed following the tragic death of her brother, Alexis struggled with care for several years before escaping to Africa. She now writes about her experience in order to promote autism acceptance, neurodiversity and to expand the biomedical conversation surrounding mental health.

First published in Great Britain 2018 by Trigger

Trigger is a trading style of Shaw Callaghan Ltd & Shaw Callaghan 23 USA, INC.

The Foundation Centre

Navigation House, 48 Millgate, Newark

Nottinghamshire NG24 4TS UK

www.triggerpublishing.com

British Library Cataloguing in Publication Data

A CIP catalogue record for this book is available upon request
from the British Library

ISBN: 978-1-912478-94-1

This book is also available in the following e-Book and Audio formats:

MOBI: 978-1-912478-97-2

EPUB: 978-1-912478-95-8

PDF: 978-1-912478-96-5

AUDIO: 978-1-912478-98-9

Cover design and typeset by Fusion Graphic Design Ltd

Printed and bound in Great Britain by Clays Ltd, Elcograf S.p.A

Paper from responsible sources

TRIGGER™

The voice of mental health

www.triggerpublishing.com

Thank you for purchasing this book.
You are making an incredible difference.

Proceeds from all Trigger books go directly to
The Shaw Mind Foundation, a global charity that focuses
entirely on mental health. To find out more about
The Shaw Mind Foundation visit,
www.shawmindfoundation.org

MISSION STATEMENT

Our goal is to make help and support available for every
single person in society, from all walks of life.
We will never stop offering hope. These are our promises.

Trigger and The Shaw Mind Foundation

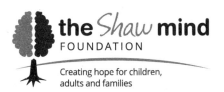

the *Shaw* mind
FOUNDATION

Creating hope for children,
adults and families

A NOTE FROM THE SERIES EDITOR

The Inspirational range from Trigger brings you genuine stories about our authors' experiences with mental health problems.

Some of the stories in our Inspirational range will move you to tears. Some will make you laugh. Some will make you feel angry, or surprised, or uplifted. Hopefully they will all change the way you see mental health problems.

These are stories we can all relate to and engage with. Stories of people experiencing mental health difficulties and finding their own ways to overcome them with dignity, humour, perseverance and spirit.

Alexis's story tells a difficult journey through misdiagnosis and consequential ill-informed treatment in the medical system. She explores what she believes is a rigid medical system in relation to people, such as herself, with neurodiversity, and talks about the adverse effects this experience has had on her. Her journey has been long and difficult, and sometimes challenging to read, but it is ultimately one of strength and survival.

This is a well-written, hard-hitting, and unique approach to mental health, one that you may have never come across before.

This is our Inspirational range. These are our stories. We hope you enjoy them. And most of all, we hope that they will educate and inspire you. That's what this range is all about.

Lauren Callaghan

Jenny Middleton and Dr David Forsythe
For seeing me, rescuing me, and setting me free.

Jaz and Dickie
For showing me how to find the road to life again, and for walking those first few steps with me before I run.

Disclaimer: Some names and identifying details have been changed to protect the privacy of individuals.

Trigger Warning: This book contains references to self-harm, sexual assault, and suicidal ideation.

Strange times are these in which we live when old and young are taught falsehoods in school. And the person that dares to tell the truth is called at once a lunatic and fool.

Plato (427 BC)

INTRODUCTION

I don't find it easy to have the courage to share with everyone what has happened to me. Yet I know that I must. I'm telling my story on behalf of the thousands of people with autism and / or learning disabilities who are inappropriately detained in hospitals for assessment and treatment, despite UK government targets for them to have been discharged by 1st June, 2014. I'm telling my story for the 85% of these who have no mental health diagnosis or behavioural risk severe enough to require treatment, but who are locked away anyway because they are easier to deal with when detained. (Health and Social Care Information Centre, 2015)[1]

We are encouraged to believe that our mental health institutions are therapeutic. The language describing their purpose supports the idea that a "service" is being provided. Yet what I experienced as a "service user" was no service. To say that psychiatry has provided me with a service is like saying a rat is a wilful consumer of rat poison.

The illusion of getting help within the mental health system was shattered for me, as I lived the unrelenting daily struggle that goes on within the walls of its institutions, which rely on the silence of people inside who cannot speak for themselves. Many are silent from fear or unable to express their needs and pose no threat to the system. Those who manage to speak out are rarely believed. I survived, and will give my account. This is my truth and my experience. It is not just about the traumatic events

I suffered in mental hospitals, but also what it felt like for me as an autistic to be confined and tortured.

I have referred to real events. To protect anonymity, I have changed some names, places, and some circumstantial details.

CHAPTER 1

Josh

Josh was my youngest brother. He was a real party animal, a very sociable kind of kid. When we were little, it felt like he had a million friends. My brother Thomas and I were never interested in that. We used to do our own stuff, play catch or have sandcastle competitions at the beach.

Josh liked to go out all the time. He lived for each day. He didn't plan, and never seemed much interested in education. Little fazed him. I often thought, *Oh, if I could have a bit of that, my life would be so much better.* For Josh, as long as he was happy in the moment, he was fine. The rest of us did the worrying for him.

He also seemed to possess a different kind of intelligence to the rest of us. He couldn't spell his last name (he always missed out an n from Quinn), but he was clever with his hands. He thatched roofs, was musically gifted, and was a complete genius on a DJ deck. He could build anything electrical as well, including cars and satellites. When Josh was little, sometimes we'd find him taking apart a TV. My mum would go nuts, but he would say, 'Don't worry, Mum, I'll put it back together when I'm done.'

'Done with what? It wasn't broken,' Mum would say.

'I know. I just wanted to see how it worked.' That was him, so inquisitive, despite the frequent shocks and mild electrocutions.

Because he was so good with his hands, Josh was always doing free repairs for his friends. This often meant that he didn't come home until late. He would come in filthy and smelly and so exhausted he would fall asleep on the couch immediately.

Every morning I would say, 'Get upstairs, Josh. You stink.'

He'd respond with, 'Lex, I had a bath two days ago and I've been busy.'

I'd say, 'Exactly! Just have a bath now. You're disgusting.'

This was how we bantered with each other. I always looked up to my little brother Josh. I loved him so much.

At two o'clock one Saturday morning, my mum woke me up and said, 'You have to come downstairs. The police are here. Something has happened with Josh.'

I came down to find two police officers in our hallway. On their radio, the dispatcher said Josh was being taken to hospital. 'It's very serious. You need to get there.'

My mum said she would look after my daughter Abi, and my dad and I would go with the police. I went upstairs to gather my things. I was fast, taking maybe less than two minutes to go up and down. When I came back, I heard on the police radio that Josh had died in transit to the hospital. I just said, 'Oh. Okay. Then maybe we should just drive in our car, and we'll see him when we get to the hospital.'

One policeman said, 'I don't think you should drive. You can come in the police car with us.'

I said, 'No, it's alright. I'll just drive because it's more convenient for when we come home.'

But they insisted, 'No, no. You really should come with us. After that news, it's not good for you to drive.' I felt somewhat disparaged – my logic was clear and had not been hijacked by my emotions the way they were implying. Yet I knew it was best not to argue with the police.

So, we went in the car with the police to the King at Heysham Hospital, K&H for short, which was nine miles from our house.

I was born in the K&H. How strange that Josh was dead there now. A nurse showed us in to see him when we got there. She said, 'I'm sorry for your loss.' I know that's a common thing to say. I've heard it in the movies, but I had a little chuckle to myself when it was said to me in real life. Films are a mirror that reflect society. I had learnt a lot from them. Here was another example. I thought about that for a few seconds.

Josh was already there lying on a bed. He looked fine to me, like when he was on the couch asleep when he came home late.

If my dad hadn't been there as well, I'd have touched Josh. But I had reasoned that conducting a scientific enquiry on a dead body, in the presence of my father and just after my little brother had died, probably wasn't in keeping with societal norms – so I didn't. I've seen dead people before, but not so close to their time of dying. He still looked alive to me. I was curious whether he was warm. I guessed he would be. I'd find out later.

*

I did the research when I got home that morning. I found the equation: 37.5°C - 1.5°C. This formula equates to the body temperature (37.5°C), which loses 1.5°C per hour until the temperature of the body is that of the environment around it, known as the ambient temperature. It may take minutes or hours to reach, depending on how cold it is. This is a good indicator of how long a body has been dead. If I had touched him then, he would've still been warm. I wish I had touched him. I wanted to feel his hair. But only on that night. Once he had been in the fridge at the funeral home, I no longer wanted to. It would have been too different. Josh was never cold. He was a warm boy.

*

We don't know the cause of Josh's death. Even after the coroner's inquest in October 2016, almost four years later. Six weeks before he died he'd gotten involved with a girl. Her friends and family had a rough reputation. He'd moved out to live with them. From that time, he was very different.

I remember on the Tuesday before he died, we were telling him we were concerned about him. He was out so often and was mixing with a different group of people. His carefree attitude had changed. When we asked him what was wrong, Josh said he was very worried because he didn't know what would happen to him. Mum said, 'Josh, just move home. We'll sort everything out.' He seemed scared. It was odd. I'd never seen him like that.

Before he died – this is from the records of the inquest – Josh collapsed and went into a seizure while he was working. An ambulance was called. There were emergency response vehicles nearby. Two drivers were reluctant to respond due to the dangerous reputation of the area Josh was in. Eventually one responded, but he wasn't a paramedic. He was an ambulance technician, the result of budget cuts. When he arrived, Josh was on the floor. There was a big puddle around him and he was having seizures. The technician quickly assessed that Josh had water in his lungs.

The driver went to get an electrical device from his bag to pump the water out of Josh. When he applied it, he realised that the battery had run out. In England, the government outsources preparation of ambulances and response gear to a private company, so the paramedics rarely check their own bags. The technician then tried to get the manual pump out of his kitbag, but he couldn't find it because the packaging had changed. It was a new device he wasn't familiar with.

As this was happening, the actual ambulance with two paramedics responded. They wanted to move Josh into the ambulance. Obviously that took time. They got him in and started resuscitation, but he died in transit to the hospital.

Dad and I arrived at the hospital a short time after Josh. Immediate blood results showed there was cocaine in his system. Because of this, it was concluded that Josh's death was not suspicious. There was no investigation of any other circumstances. The crime scene was allowed to disintegrate, so there was never any evidence gathered to find out what had happened. They just picked him up, put him in the ambulance, and that was that.

Some of Josh's friends were at the hospital that night. These big, rough and ready guys were crying. I found myself consoling them. We spoke with them and the police, and then we went home.

Josh died on 1st December, 2012. He was 24.

CHAPTER 2

Family

My parents started to manage my differences quite early. At 10 months, I was tearing around Tesco's supermarket to the delighted squeals of neighbours. Seemingly focused and determined right from the start, I was able to swim 25 metres at the age of one. Day and night, I didn't stop moving. My worried mother took me to the doctor at the age of three because I never slept. She explained to him, 'I come down in the night to Lexi singing nursery rhymes and jumping on the bed. She does forward rolls around the room. What is with her?'

The doctor just said, 'Exercise her.'

Children were not labelled with autism or ADHD so readily in the 1980s – I was told I was just different and the prescription was exercise. The health visitor who came to check on me just thought I was naughty. She told my mum that I needed better discipline. One day when my mother and I were in Tesco's and I was having a meltdown in the aisle, Mum saw the health visitor there. I was on my back with my legs in the air, screaming. She asked the health visitor to demonstrate to her, and the crowd watching, how to "help" me. The visitor failed. From that moment on, my mum raised me her own way.

I consider myself very lucky to have my supportive family and appreciative parents. I'm autistic, and my family is far from "the normal". I lack awareness of many of my own emotions, but I'm the daughter of a warm, cuddly mother. I am logical – most emotional states do not influence my judgement – yet I'm the daughter of a free-thinking and creative father.

My older brother Sean, who lives in Liverpool, was born during my dad's first marriage. He has always lived with his mother. My mum and dad met when Sean was just three or four years old. Soon after they married, they had me, then Thomas, then Josh. The three of us grew up in a five-bedroomed house in a small coastal town in England.

Our house was Victorian, old but well looked-after. Each room had an open fireplace, so they were warm and full of character. Family photos adorned the walls, showing affection and pride in our achievement. Life has always offered plenty to celebrate and much to overcome in the Quinn family.

As I aged, I struggled and was bullied at school. I was unusually academic, very athletic but socially awkward. However, I wasn't seen as defective or broken but simply eccentric, sometimes brilliant and rarely inappropriate.

Academia became a place where I could immerse myself in knowledge. Nothing less than the best grades and a first-class honours degree from Edinburgh University would do. The bar was set high when I was young. I had an exceptional, almost eidetic memory, and there were expectations to perform, from both my parents and me.

I can recall patterns, numbers, and images for a long time after I've seen them. I didn't know that I was unique in doing this. I've tried using this skill to my advantage as a party trick, charming a few blokes in the past with facts I could recall. Predictably, this has rarely been successful. If important enough, I can remember strings of conversation and text, which I see as patterns on a page. This, I learnt, was more useful in school than trying to be charming.

I didn't have many friends growing up. I picked up one or two a year while I was working overseas. I picked up a few during my time as a confined person in the mental health system. You get to know people very well when you're locked up with them 24 / 7 for years. Now my friend count is fairly normal for someone my age. And they usually stick around for the long haul.

I have little drama in my friendships. What you see is what you get with me. Rarely aware of my own emotions, I can listen well when presented with a problem. I can be reasonable, open-minded, and objectively sceptical, and as a result I am often the friend people depend on not to judge or gossip.

I guess I could tell from a young age that I was never going to be Miss Popular, and it didn't bother me much.

Thomas, Josh, and I all grew to over six feet tall, and we're naturally very athletic. I spent forever in the pool when my head wasn't in a book. What I missed in social learning with friends, I made up for in family activities.

We weren't rich but I never felt that I was in want of anything. The greatest gift my parents gave me was their time. My mum and dad took the exercise thing very seriously. I guess they had to, to modulate my expressions of hyperactivity and impulsivity. I did five to seven sports a week until I was about eight years old, including gymnastics, judo, swimming, and a load of team games. Poor Thomas and Josh had to do them too. I remember both my brothers in their little gymnastic leotards late into their primary school years. Mum and Dad became our taxi service.

I cherished our time together. Our garden was little but it contained pleasing natural stuff like bricks and sand. Thomas and I would spend a lot of time in the garden, throwing tennis balls, trying to hit a brick from over 10 metres away. Meanwhile, Josh would be out with his friends. I'm glad I had one brother to keep me company.

Routine was majorly important in our household, as we had to keep a tight schedule with all our activities. My dad was also ritualistic about things like table manners. He would say, 'Lexi, your drink must be on the right side of your plate, in line with your dessert spoon,' or 'Josh, I've told you to eat with your mouth closed,' and 'Thomas, if you put your elbows on the table again, you will be in trouble.' It gave a sense of knowing and also belonging. Things were always the same and we knew what to expect.

My mum remained a bog-standard police officer for her 34 years in the police. My dad's jobs weren't that well paid. He was in the army, then a prison officer, and he worked in schools later in his life. We lived from month to month but I consider us to have been rich in family.

Commitment is a value I learnt young. In my family, it was based on trust and respect – putting family first. Sport drained our finances; swim suits were over a hundred pounds apiece (for a racing suit), petrol for the 15-mile round trip to the swimming pool we attended twice a day, the galas I attended which required hotel stays for the national and international trip meets. These were just the basic expenses for the life I was living.

Thomas and I were both swimmers. We both competed for Great Britain in swimming and Thomas achieved world champion status in another sport. When I was 15, I moved to Scotland on my own to join the new national swimming academy until I was injured three years later. My injury was in both elbows and was chronic. It ended my career in sport as a competitor completely. Until 2002, my special interest was swimming. For many years I made it my business to know everything I could. I collected different goggles, swimming hats, and memorised timings of past Olympians. I systematically searched for the lesser-known details, and built theories about best practices that hadn't been thought of before. I was a water expert.

Josh was different from Thomas and I. He dropped out of sport as soon as he could put a reasoned argument to my parents. He was different also, with various neurodevelopmental labels, as was my older brother Sean. They struggled in school and didn't do well. But they were differently able. Both Josh and Sean were good with their hands. They could fix anything.

My mum, although sometimes frustrated, always let Josh, Thomas, and I express ourselves in our own ways.

Heavily invested in our achievement, my parents would drive us to London sometimes for specialist training. On the journey, we talked the whole way. I'd discuss things I had learnt and current interests I had. I found the English language a real fascination. Did you know that the word "alphabet" comes from the Greek words alpha and beta, and that 'e' is the most common letter in the English language? For every eight letters written, one is an 'e'. I know a lot of useless but interesting stuff. My parents accepted this about me and encouraged me to pursue my interests. They would talk to me and listen. And not just listen in the way parents sometimes do, but actually listen. They never quietened my mind or my mouth as I discussed my facts with them. I realise now that this helped me to make conversation and mask my poor receptive language.

I learnt expressive communication from keen observation and study. Always confident, I have spoken in public since primary school. I don't get anxious and I'm good at copying non-verbal cues from inspirational speakers. Language usage can mostly be learnt. I'm useless at puns, but I know how they work. Most words are ambiguous. Our brains quickly grasp the right meaning from context. People understand puns when they know multiple meanings of a word. For example, when the Beatles were asked, 'How did you find America?', John responded, 'Turn left at Greenland.' Many autistics wouldn't get the joke.

My family is strong. We were able to manage stress and crisis, and overcome hardships together. We have always worked together rather than pulling apart. We've been tested beyond anything we could have imagined. With all we've been through, we're different now. Crisis can be an opportunity to help each other. But the difficulties I will tell you about broke us and we couldn't all come back.

CHAPTER 3

Abidemi

My daughter Abi was born in March 2012. Her father is a Nigerian tech guy in the school where I worked. We were together for a short time before I got pregnant. When he found out I was pregnant, that pretty much ended the relationship. I named her Abidemi, which in Nigeria means "child born during father's absence".

I found the pregnancy to be quite stressful. Too many body changes, changes in my life circumstances, and people wanting to touch my belly! I had to leave home 15 minutes early so I could walk to work instead of run. My life was no longer focused on just me. Now it had to include the small thing I was growing inside me. Not that I was selfish. It was just such a huge adaptation to make in a life focused on maintaining my status quo.

When I was pregnant, I felt weird and different. I couldn't enjoy my pregnancy. But you can't say that to people. I was in Asia surfing and wake boarding, doing all kinds of sports. When I realised that I must change my routine and let go of the extreme sports, I thought, *Do I have to have this baby? How will I manage without my usual activities?* I thought I should not want to not have a baby because I would rather go surfing. But I sorely missed my surfing friends. *Why am I so averse to change,* I wondered?

Why am I not excited about this? These thoughts dominated my thinking, right or wrong, when I found out I was pregnant.

I'd been teaching in Asia and hadn't planned to leave. I intended to bring up Abi overseas, and hoped to sort things out with her daddy. I'm a person who always has a five-year life plan. I flew home to give birth just so she would have a British passport. When she was old enough to fly, I was going to go back to Asia. At home in England, in anticipation of the year later when my contract expired, I put out loads of CVs.

A grammar school phoned me up and said, 'Can you come for an interview? Can you come on Monday, 6th March?'

I told them, 'Actually, that's my due date.'

'Oh,' they said. 'You're having a baby. But we need you to start in five weeks.' I wasn't expecting that.

I said, 'That's fine, because I would've been flying to Asia then anyway.' I would save a year in my five-year plan. So I called my employers and told them I wasn't coming back. They weren't very happy. Then I started my new job, in a grammar school in Kingshire when Abi was five weeks old. I was lucky to have the part-time position, teaching wonderful girls just a few hours a day.

CHAPTER 4

How I Became "Mad"

December 2012

Josh was pronounced dead by Dr Adbullah at 1.50am. I went to the gym at six o'clock in the morning. I did my scheduled one-hour class in Heysham, which was nine miles from my house. Then I went for a swim and came back, business as usual. Everyone at home seemed sad. They were crying. I wasn't. They were talking about Josh. I wasn't. They wanted unscheduled human connection and company. I did not. I started to notice that I was different and those around me told me how I was. I tried harder to "fit in".

Over the next few days, I was busy organising the funeral with Thomas. It was just like I was organising a swim meet at school. I was meticulous. I took care of all the invitations and designed a cool coffin with amazing graphics on it. I was proud of that. Everyone liked it. It was a true reflection of all Josh's loves in life. The coffin was a gradient of blue – dark blue at the bottom of the coffin that became lighter towards the top. We drew Josh's first and most loved car on two sides of the coffin as a cartoon. He had modified a Ford Escort XR3i which he did in a boy racer style – all of his modifications were accounted for in our graphic depiction. On the other side of the coffin was a cartoon scuba diver as Josh loved diving and spent years overseas teaching.

On the top of the coffin were musical symbols to depict his love of music. We captured everything.

When I was organising, I was fine. I had about a fortnight's rest before I was like, 'Damn, where is he?' When I came down in the morning, Josh wasn't on the couch. With my familiar routine gone, I became lost.

I had seen a Mother and Infant Mental Health Service, MIMHS, psychiatrist, Dr Nowak, to monitor the ADHD drug I was taking. I had taken this drug since I was 18 when I was diagnosed by a private psychiatrist due to problems I was having at university. I told her that Josh had died. She said, 'Oh, your brother died.' She thought I was acting peculiarly so she got a crisis team involved.

A crisis resolution and home treatment team is a group of mental health professionals who support you at your home during a mental health crisis. They have a lot of professionals in the team like psychiatrists, social workers, nurses, and support workers. Mostly I saw support workers and the occasional nurse.

When Josh was in the funeral parlour, a two-minute walk around the corner from our house, I would see him every day. I thought, *I won't be able to see him soon so I need to make the most of this.* I liked to look at him. For the first few days he looked fine. But after a while I noticed the way his body was decaying. His eyes got a lot more sunken. His face looked stretched.

I found it interesting. That's when I started reading about decay. Death and statistics became my special interest. The mental health professionals would ask me how I was. I said, 'I read some interesting information about physiological responses to decay.'

Because of Josh's death, I was again reminded of how "weird" I was. How people respond to death is learnt. I had not practised grieving. My only knowledge of how to act was in offering condolences. In England, a certain amount of empathy is required, and unwritten rules should be followed. 'I'm sorry for your loss,' I would say. I was good at that. But when it's your brother, this isn't appropriate. Nor is it okay to say, 'It's okay' when someone offers you sympathy. I learnt that pretty quickly. These unwritten rules vary from person to person based on the degree of emotional impact I needed to express. I wasn't comfortable with the procedures around comforting, crying together, flowers, and reminiscing. I had read an article about Charles Darwin, who said that emotional tears were "purposeless". I agree. Did you know that humans are the only creatures whose tears can be triggered by their feelings?

My family was housing an ever-growing collection of flowers and hosting a continuous stream of people. The flower thing seemed like a colossal waste of money. Flowers are just hard work: they stink and the scents of the different bouquets clash with one another. They require a lot of care, from the initial unwrapping, to cutting the bottoms of the stocks, which are slimy, to putting them in a vase, which gets dirty, and then feeding them. A few days later they die – a pointless waste of money and time. The whole idea of creating more work for somebody who has already had their life turned upside down makes no sense.

Everyone told me that I was handling Josh's death well. This wasn't true. Can you imagine?

How are you, Lexi?

Well, I feel rather uncomfortable about the whole thing, really.

This is not what you say, I knew that much. But I said it to Dr Nowak, the Mother and Infant's Mental Health doctor. I could be honest with her.

I hated people's changing emotional states. One minute we would be going shopping, and the next I had to console my mum. When they'd reach out to hug me, I knew that if I turned away that would make things worse, and we'd never get to go out, so I obliged. I didn't want to touch Mum, or anyone for that matter – especially with all the tears and snot generated from a lengthy cry. I had thought about getting a broom and using that to stroke her back from a distance. I didn't, obviously.

Compared to my brother's friends and my family, I was rational, logical, and made it my mission to be organised. This was the best approach to have a decent funeral timeline. They couldn't go shopping on time or walk the dog at the normal hour, so I had little faith in their ability to organise a big event. Unlike me, Josh had lots of friends, and they all wanted to see him off.

Because it was Christmas, there was no school, no fitness classes at the gym, and no baby groups. I found this hard because I liked to know what I was doing and when. When I tried to create structure for myself, I would be interrupted by someone coming to the house to grieve with us or by my family's own grieving. This always involved cancelling plans. It was chaos.

A friend bought me a book on the grieving process. I thought my process must have skipped right to the end of the phases, because I couldn't relate to any of them. I started to run again and felt immediately better. The constant movement made my head less busy.

I became averse to everything that related to Josh which affected my routine. When I'd wake in the morning, I usually looked in the front room to see if he was lying there. Knowing he wouldn't be there, I avoided looking in the front room at all. I didn't want to open the fridge where I could now drink the milk – he hadn't been slurping out of it. I didn't like to enter the bathroom which was clean for once. Daily routines became difficult to avoid and so I experienced major discomfort as I went about my day.

People told me that it had been only two weeks and I obviously needed more time to come to terms with what happened. *More time for what?* I thought. Josh was dead. It seemed I was coming up short in the empathy department. Our dogs seemed better able to read emotions than I did. I, a two-legged sister of the deceased, had such great difficulty recognising not only how the people around me were feeling, but also how I felt.

I was sure my feelings were there somewhere. I would consciously check in to see what they were up to, usually after someone had asked me how I was. I was always at the ready with the *right* answer. Or at least what I thought was the right answer – this answer was as sought after as gold dust to me. What I would have given to know the best things to say.

But I wasn't thinking feelings, I was feeling them in my body – this was strange. I could tell no one except Dr Nowak. She would understand. I realised that I wasn't lacking focus. I was focusing just fine. That's why I could do research. It was hyper-focus, a type of sensitivity. I couldn't process as I had before. Or I was processing, but I was doing it too much. And I couldn't stop.

The worst was when I was driving. I would count the lines on the road in the day and the lamp posts by night. This wasn't easy at 70 mph. At the start of junctions on the motorway, I liked to know the first number stamped on the lamp post. I don't know why, but it felt reassuring. I hadn't done this before.

Days passed, and this hyper-focus was getting worse. It was very exhausting and annoying.

Sight and sound started to become overbearing. Having not experienced sensory sensitivity before to this degree, I craved silence. This was hard with a baby. I felt like a terrible parent. Thankfully, my mum and dad looked after Abi when I was out running. Abi was quite a helpful distraction for them. When I ran, things eased, so I ran more and more. I found I loved the sound of traffic and white noise so I ran next to main roads.

I did not understand what was happening to me, but it was clear some things helped and others didn't. Going out to shops, which was challenging enough before my life was upturned, was to be avoided at all cost. I could only last 10–20 minutes. I couldn't find items on the shelves. The sound of the trolleys and the poor acoustics meant that by the time I got to the checkout, I really needed to leave. But then I was bombarded with the beeping of all the registers scanning everyone's items. I could hardly stop myself from screaming out.

I thought I was going insane. I tried to stay focused on what helped – running and my special interest. Everything else I avoided. I became more reclusive. Not because I didn't like people, but because it was way too hard. I couldn't respond to what people said because I couldn't process quickly with a good-enough answer. I had to wear loose-fitting clothing. My skin felt like pins and needles when people touched me – but only when I was feeling too much of the "something" inside me.

These changes made me very anxious. And the more anxious I became, the worse the symptoms were. I wanted to find the cause, but nothing I read about grief pointed to anything like this. Worse, too, was that nothing I read about anxiety, depression, or any physical ailment could be identified for my changes. I was soon in a perpetual cycle of anxiety / symptoms. When I spoke to the crisis team and Dr Nowak, I wanted their plan of reasonable, intelligent suggestions and actions to help me.

I got more drugs instead.

I knew I was struggling. My stress made processing how I was feeling about the death impossible. I was consumed by worry about my "weirdness". This worsened my reactions and I withdrew into myself. I was filled with panic. My environment, always the same, was now horrifically out of control. When I tried to make a plan, it was thwarted. I was scared all day as I had to meander through constant surprises and people shattering my sense of inner calm. I realised my life was completely interrupted by this shocking event. I was so obsessed that the death itself was never foremost in my mind.

I was sick of hearing, 'I just can't believe it'. I would think to myself, *Well, believe it, because he's dead – I saw it with my own eyes*. Why were these intelligent people telling me they couldn't believe something as real as death? Society dictates that when the funeral is over, the mourning is over. I had not yet begun. People stepped in to help me by "being there". This made it worse. I was antisocial. Never mind that being around people was making my head explode and my skin burn. My stance was only seen as rudeness and indifference.

Also, I was very confused about the growing oddities of my sensory world. My information processing had become disturbed. Patterns formed everywhere I looked. My hearing was so sensitive. My skin tingled. Eating was very unpleasant. When I put food in my mouth, it was like a mouthful of sandy stones from the beach. The food was so heavy I had to change my diet, and cut down on what I was eating to avoid being sick.

The strangest thing I noticed about myself was this new curiosity about death. I became highly interested in it. How did Josh die? What happened to him medically? And why on earth did it take 17 days to get a funeral date? It turns out December is quite a popular month in which to die. I researched types of death, death rate, average age of death, and quickly became obsessed with the numbers.

*

In the funeral room, the walls were beige and the carpet plain. It was an okay place. It was quiet. The smell I had to contend with, but once I knew what it was I found it interesting. Pungent flowers were in a corner, and the pong of embalming fluid emanated from the cadaver. Associating such a smell with Josh was a bit weird. I didn't mind it though. After the first two visits, I had learnt that embalming fluid contained many disinfectant agents, preservatives, and additives such as formaldehyde, glutaraldehyde, and methanol.

The science of it was most fascinating. The fluid denatures cellular proteins, stopping them acting as a nutrient source for bacteria. I was pleased Josh was being cremated because I didn't want him to be overcome by bacteria. Interestingly, Josh didn't change colour that much. You may be surprised to find it was due to the formaldehyde, which fixes the cells by irreversibly connecting a primary amine group in a protein molecule with nearby nitrogen in a DNA molecule through a – CH_2 linkage. Clever stuff.

The walls had faint marks of dirt on them. Sometimes, when I went to see Josh, they wouldn't bother me. Other times they stood out big and bold as if they were drawn in a permanent marker. Nobody else noticed them. This pattern forming was happening all the time now.

I established that the dots on the wall mostly resembled Ophiuchus, a star constellation. I told no one, as I told no one about my death research – except Dr Nowak. She would understand. Wherever I looked, I would tell her, I could see constellations. This strange thing started happening after Josh died. I explained that the constellation Serpentarius in the funeral home on the north wall is commonly represented as a man grasping a snake. It is one of 88 modern constellations northwest of the centre of the Milky Way. It was very settling for me, as where it was in the room was accurate from a navigation perspective, opposite Orion in the sky.

Galileo used the appearance of a supernova found in Ophiuchus to counter the Aristotelian dogma that the heavens are changeless. The heavens were constantly changing and so was my world, so I was pleased that I could calm my visual world with constellations. I became an expert – Dr Nowak said little about that.

I'd lie on my bed looking at the ceiling and the constellation Lyra would jump out at me. I could see its main asterism of six stars. The other 73 stars weren't in the right place on my ceiling (obviously), which was frustrating. However, I arranged a few of the luminous stars you can buy to make the constellation work better. Especially the star called Vega, because it's the brightest and best known in the constellation. Astronomers call Vega the most important star after the sun, so I used the biggest luminous star to mark its place.

As the funeral plans were finalised, I lost the structure it had provided. When Josh was cremated I could no longer visit him every day. Another routine lost. This is when things began to get bad. I needed to isolate myself in a low-sensory room so I could process and problem-solve my thoughts. But I couldn't – I had a baby and a façade of regularity to maintain.

Rainy weather was a massive issue I had to deal with when trying to maintain my essential routine of running. During regular rain (5 mm across / house fly size), which falls at 20 mph, I felt like I was being pelted with hail stones. When the rain was light and faint (0.5 mm across), falling at 4.5 mph, it was like having a tattoo. Running became intolerable. My skin was too sensitive. Although the monotony of the rhythmic plod-plod-plod was calming, the rain had to be avoided. So, I created an early-morning routine of checking the weather forecast to ensure I earmarked the best hours to go. This was considerably more efficient. Various rules were created around this routine. I had to run only numbers of minutes that were multiples of six. I could only start my run at specific times.

When running, I passed by many patterns / constellations. As the run progressed, my brain seemed to relax and rest. By the end I could experience the environment as usual. If I did a long run, I would return home not seeing anything unusual.

One day, not long after the funeral, I had to meet my friend Roxi at a café on the sea front. She thought she was helping, and her mum was an old friend of my mum. They wanted us to meet up – to get me out of the house, I expect. I wasn't very enthused because I knew the sound would be overwhelming (groups of people talking, doors opening and closing, chairs moving), and most likely my ears would hurt. I was distressed just thinking about it. Plus, the extended physical contact would make my skin hurt. The visual overstimulation meant I would spend the whole time trying to unsee patterns no one else could see. And I knew I wouldn't be able to see her without running first.

I went for a huge two-hour run before the meet-up time. I arrived three minutes early so I could find a good place to sit, but it was so busy there were few tables. Roxi was quite late, about 10 minutes, as she had to pick up her son from school. Her lateness, combined with the surprise of her son being there, threw me. When Roxi turned up, she grimaced as she ran her eyes over my sweat-covered body. She didn't shake my hand or give me hug – result! Nor did I feel like she really wanted to be sitting with me.

The question I hated most was, 'How do you feel?' I didn't know, and had no idea what to answer. I was told that if I cried it would help. I tried, but I never could cry about Josh. I was getting closer to understanding how he physiologically might have died. I knew death is caused by a cascading failure of interdependent systems. Since I didn't know the cause of his death, I couldn't work out where the cascading failure began and how the failure spread in such a way to make organism recovery impossible. This caused a feeling inside me which was very unpleasant.

The maternal health doctor would ask me what I'd been doing to help myself cope with Josh's death. She didn't appreciate my desire to know the exact order of his system failure. I didn't know what to do after that.

Apparently how I was coping was wrong.

So, after a while I told her I cried. She seemed pleased because she smiled at me. I thought that rather inappropriate. She asked me how it felt. I said it made me feel hot, wet, and my eyes stung for a while. She laughed at me. I thought she was very rude. What did she want me to say? First she insults my relief strategies, which I thought were very good, and then she laughs at how I cry. What is the right answer? She wasn't helping much.

*

I made a table about my "changes" and what helped:

Changes	Things that help
Worry	Looking at the time
Feeling uncomfortable all the time	Being alone
Hyper-focus	Spending time researching death
Obsessive about patterns and numbers	Researching common causes of death in men
Cannot respond to people easily	Running more than two hours a day
Can't hear things outside / too noisy	Lifting weights
Don't like to be touched	Initiate a handshake to avoid a hug
Clothes feel prickly / pins and needles	Wear loose clothing
I am weird compared to others	Focusing on my needs and not comparing myself to others – which was hard as everyone was doing it

*

Kingshire police were refusing to investigate Josh's death, so there were still many questions. As I researched for elusive answers to my healthy brother's sudden passing, my enthusiasm was seen as a disturbed obsession and mental illness. Yet I felt a sense of closure as I learnt how Josh's body most likely shut down.

Have you ever wondered what you will die from? I hadn't, and now I needed to know so I could be prepared. My favourite study was the 2010 data from Reddit by UCanDoEat, created by the Institute of Health Metrics and Evaluation. This provided statistics on the most common causes. Transport injuries (36%) and suicide (29–32%) are the leading causes of death for young people. As people age, cancer and other diseases arise but astonishingly, intentional harm and mental illness account for a significant portion of deaths at nearly every age. Wow. People died intentionally ... *How strange*, I remember thinking. I had not assumed that would be a leading cause. And so began my obsession with suicide.

My research relaxed me ... but got me labelled as mentally ill.

CHAPTER 5

Crisis Team

I lost so much weight after Josh died. I was 84 kilograms and went down to 61. I could eat nothing. Every time I put food in my mouth it felt as though I had swallowed stones from the beach. When I did force food into my mouth I was sick. I was trying to be fine for Abi, but it was impossible.

It was after the funeral, on the 17th December, when the crisis team came. I must've looked particularly terrible. They said, 'You're really not looking good, Alexis.' The Crisis Team gets involved when you're in a mental health crisis. As the name suggests, they give urgent help to people who have a mental health problem and who are considered high risk. I wasn't in a crisis and I didn't identify as having a mental health problem. At that time, I thought I was fine. I was struggling, though, because lots of things weren't the same.

I couldn't stop wondering why my brother wasn't there, and why he had died. When mental health services asked me questions about how I was managing or coping, I told them about my research, blissfully unaware of the alarm it was causing them. I didn't know they found it troubling and an indication of "illness". I thought they were interested. I am unable to think what others might be thinking about what I am thinking. The crisis team visits were in some ways contributing to the crisis.

They'd phone me in the morning and say, 'We are coming to visit you today.'

I'd ask, 'What time are you coming?'

They'd say, 'We don't know.' Or, 'We will let you know.'

Sometime later I'd phone them. 'Okay, I need to know what time you're coming. I'm waiting in.'

They'd just say, 'We'll be there soon.'

By late afternoon I'd phone them and say, 'I've waited in the whole day. Where are you?'

'Oh, we're coming. We've been busy.'

'What time tonight?' I always went to bed at six o'clock so I could try to sleep from six o'clock to ten o'clock. My mum and dad looked after Abi so I could have a four-hour block of sleep. But Abi wasn't a sleeper. She would breastfeed for 45 minutes and fall asleep. Then it would take me 15 minutes to get to sleep. An hour and a half later she'd wake up. So I was on a two-hour cycle. I'd get an hour and 15 minutes while she was asleep and then I'd have to do it all again.

I told them, 'I can't see you from six o'clock to ten o'clock.'

'Well, we'll come after that.'

'No, I want to try to sleep.'

'We're here to help you, Alexis.'

One time they rang the doorbell at two o'clock. We have two big boxer dogs, who would bark their heads off. I carried Abi downstairs. Everyone in the house would wake up. The team stayed for 10 or 15 minutes, checking that I was still alive, and then they left.

I saw them daily until I went into hospital on 24th December.

The crisis team said, 'We think you should go into hospital for a rest.'

I said, 'Yes, I'm very stressed. I have a baby, a job, and my brother's dead.'

Perhaps I did need a rest.

CHAPTER 6

Incarcerated in the NHS

24th December 2012

Okay, I'll go, I decided. So, Mum drove me to Blackthorn hospital in Kingshire and I was admitted to Clover Ward. It was 9 miles from our house in Morecombe Cove. We went in there, and it was like a scene out of *One Flew Over the Cuckoo's Nest.* The corridors felt narrow, nowhere to move, and dimly lit. When you enter the ward, you face a large glass office that faces on to the corridor door. I approached the desk, but to speak to the nurse, I had to bend down, open a little hatch and talk through that. It was undignified. I felt I couldn't be trusted to have a normal conversation. It made me cross when I first went there.

Mum and I were sitting waiting for someone to admit me. We were waiting for about 30 minutes. I hoped we could perhaps talk through a plan. Get things straight in my mind. Understand my new world. I thought, *Maybe they can help me with that.*

Finally, a health care assistant (HCA), came to admit me. She asked my height, whether I had any tattoos, smoked, took drugs – mundane questions like that. I was thinking, *Why is this relevant?* While I was with the HCA, my mum was watching what was going on in the ward. She would later tell me:

There was a little, old lady in one room. She had a member of staff watching her all the time. This was Christmas Day and her husband had been to visit. The couple looked very professional. The lady was probably in her mid-70s. As soon as the husband left, this member of staff sitting outside her room said to her, 'Headmistress. Headmistress. What would the children think of you now? Look at the state of you.' The old woman got up and went absolutely crazy. Then he pressed the alarm and all hell let loose. Nurses came and restrained her, threw her in the bed, said, 'Don't you touch her,' to the staff member. This took about half an hour. No sooner had they gone than he started it again to her. 'Headmistress, Headmistress.'

I couldn't believe what my mum told me. We said nothing to anyone then. My mum reported it later, though.

There were people with vacant expressions standing and shuffling from foot to foot. Some paced the corridors. One woman was talking to herself and moving around pieces of fruit like action figures in a child's game. Many were shouting and swearing. An alarm sounded at one point and I didn't know if it was a fire alarm. People were coming and going from the locked doors.

I knew this wasn't the place for me. This was not helping. But where was the place for me? *At least here I might get the help I need,* I thought. Panic was setting in.

So, I said to staff, 'I want to leave. Thank you.'

They said, 'I'm sorry, but you can't leave.'

I said, 'Well, I can, so you need to let me out the door now, or at least let me go for a walk because I need some space.' I was really sleep deprived, and I wanted my child. I was still breast-feeding. This was another painful thing because Abi wasn't taking milk so I was uncomfortable. So, I said, 'You need to let me out now,' and they wouldn't. I felt a rush of emotion inside me. I was fuming that I couldn't get out, and panicked because I was stuck in this oppressive unit with too much going on.

They took me into a room and put me on a Section 5(4). I didn't know what the hell a Section 5(4) was. I found out it's known as the nurse's holding power. This can only be used when you must be immediately stopped from leaving hospital for your own health or safety or for protecting others, or if it's not possible to get a doctor who can section you under the doctor's holding power, Section 5(2), for 72 hours.

The deputy ward manager, Jeremy, told me they were holding me because I was an unknown. He said, 'Most people in this ward we've known for years.'

I told him, 'I have no intention of staying here for years. I want to leave right now. I don't want to get to know you. I don't want you to know me. I don't want to have anything to do with this place. You need to let me out.'

He said, 'No.' I learnt that he is supposed to explain my rights and what the section involves but staff rarely have the time to do that. Jeremy explained that on a 5(4) if the doctor doesn't show up within six hours, I can leave. I saw no doctors there, so I thought, *Maybe they won't come.* That occupied my mind while I watched the seconds, minutes, and hours tick by.

After five-and-a-half hours, I felt sure the doctor wasn't coming, because nobody had turned up.

Then the doctor came. He told me I couldn't leave, and was being put on a Section 5(2) because there was no consultant psychiatrist on shift. I lost it. I said, 'You rapscallion! You have to let me out!' But I was held there for 72 hours. On Monday, I think it was, the psychiatrist came in. She interviewed me and discharged me.

Trigger Warning: This chapter contains references to self-harm.

CHAPTER 7

Quetiapine

15th January 2013

There were no beds available in Heysham. But they phoned around and found me a bed in a Priory Hospital. The Priory is a group of private hospitals. My only knowledge of them was of the exclusive Priory in London, where the rich and famous people go. The crisis team told Mum and me the available bed was in Hove, a two-hour drive from our family home. We had to get ourselves there. So, I said goodbye to Abi, and off I went to Hove.

This Priory was wonderful. We were greeted by a nurse. She was in her 40s, well dressed, and so respectful and kind.

She said, 'I think we can really help you. We read your history and we think we can help you. It will involve a few hours of therapy a day. We have a new Cognitive Behavioural Therapy, CBT, cycle starting.'

I was there for one week. In that time, I learnt that CBT was used to change the way I thought and behaved in relation to my problems. I realised during this stay I had no problems with the way I thought about things or the way I behaved. I understood that it was others who had the problems with me. I felt even more weird and worried. On the bright side, it was helpful thinking about what had happened and talking about it in a systematic way.

Later, it would occur to me that I had been there on Josh's birthday, January 20.

The Priory was a lovely place because the days ran on routines. It was quiet and the atmosphere felt healing. There were other professional people like me talking about what was going on with them. It was busy, but in a calm way, and it was stimulating in a healing way. The food was also amazing.

On my seventh day at the Priory, I was recalled to the NHS.

*

Dr Nowak had prescribed me the drug quetiapine. I began having thoughts about, and researching, suicide. I spent hours thinking how one might go about it. I didn't think I would do it. I just obsessed about it. I didn't want to die, but I was very curious about how the different methods actually worked. As my dose of the cocktail of drugs increased, these thoughts became stronger and stronger.

On Josh's birthday, I made a small cut on my arm. As a result, I was put on a more intrusive observation. This was my first time on observations or obs for short. I found out there are different kinds. There is the 1:1, where a member of staff watches you constantly. There is a 2:1, where there are two people watching you. Then there is arms-length, which means you can't be any more than arm's distance from the observer. In Priory, I was on 1:1. Although obs are intrusive, staff were very respectful and it was fine.

I was troubled by my cutting and was deeply embarrassed. In the tranquillity of the Priory unit, where I had the space and time to reflect, I thought about what I had done to myself. It was a big deal for me. I didn't know why I did it. It seemed so pointless, yet the desire to cut was strong. I looked it up: 'Why do people cut?' I then analysed my action using the top three reasons people self-harm according to my research:

1. It didn't take away any emotional pain. Actually, it added to it as now I felt ashamed.
2. It didn't stop me feeling numb. Actually, it caused me to analyse, analyse, analyse. I felt numb all the time anyway. I felt little emotion – that was normal for me.
3. It wasn't an alternative outlet for emotional pain. I actually got to talk a lot in Priory and that was the only outlet I needed then.

So why did I do it? All it had done was cause a situation where this guy had to watch me continually. I also will have a horrible scar on my arm that I'll have to explain to anyone who sees it.

*

For months, no one recognised the effect of the drug on me. That April, Mum and Dad flew to the United States on holiday. There they saw all the drug adverts on TV. In the UK, we're not such a Pharma nation. We don't see these ads, and we don't talk about mental health so much.

My mum said to the family, 'Oh, my gosh. This drug causes agitation, self-harm, and suicidal thoughts.' When my parents came home they were telling everyone, 'This is what's happening to Alexis.' But nobody would listen because I was lost by that stage.

CHAPTER 8

Beginning of Poor Treatment and Abuse

23rd January 2013

I was recalled from the Priory to the NHS. I kept saying I didn't want to go. My mum came to pick me up and she asked Priory staff if there was any way my family could pay for me to stay. They said because I had self-harmed and was on 1:1 obs, the cost would be out of our price range.

I was so deflated about having to leave. My family would have had enough money if I hadn't harmed myself. I felt I could have gotten better at the Priory. I'd been having about four hours of therapy every day and plenty of informal input. The Priory in Hove was well staffed with clinicians who spent time with their patients.

I was sent back to a poxy Blackthorn hospital. The brand-new ward I was on was called Primrose. I guess the modern look caused me to have some hope when I arrived. It was spacious inside, with natural light. The furniture was new. There was a large courtyard measuring about 30 metres by 20 metres. At the other side of the ward was a smaller garden. I expected a calm, therapeutic environment where people spoke to you, where people listened to why you were there and tried to help. Soon, I realised it was an aesthetically pleasing bedlam.

People were very distressed and some were obviously seeing and hearing things. Occasionally people would kick off. This was usually in response to "needs not being met", which was the way the staff put it. For example, if the staff didn't allow for a cigarette break, that would rile people up.

The ward and its occupants smelt terrible. Some were homeless and awaiting housing. Many people didn't bathe. I noticed early on that self-awareness was a luxury for those with enough energy and well-being to pay attention to it. When you are in such distress and it's hard to even get out of bed, the last thing you're worried about is brushing your teeth. When you are so tired from contemplating harming yourself and feel like giving up entirely, you aren't likely to prioritise a bath.

When I arrived at Primrose, I was still an informal patient. This meant I could leave any time – if they let me out. I went into this ward expecting them to carry on unravelling why on earth this was happening. But they didn't do that. They hardly even spoke to me. I was shown my room and given the key card to open it. That was it.

The room was a good size. The bed was a block bolted to the floor with a blue waterproof mattress on it. There was an adjacent en-suite bathroom and a shelved wardrobe without a door.

My first few days were disturbing, to say the least. I was scared. Not only of myself and my own dysregulation and vulnerability, but also because I was suddenly locked in with other people in conditions of such distress I had not known existed. The airlock was a space of about 10 metres with a set of locked double doors at each end. There was no escaping our madness.

I reflected that I had been so closeted by my privileged life that I was segregated from an important slice of humanity. But I am embarrassed to admit that I was thinking, *What has happened that I find myself here?* The NHS had been paying for me to have treatment in a helpful place, with like-minded people. Now there was no treatment and no one I could relate to.

*

I wanted to go out.

Staff said, 'You can't go out. You can go in the courtyard.'

So, I said, 'Fine. Just let me in the courtyard.' This is when I realised the value of pacing without picking up on the anxieties it caused staff.

They said, 'You seem to be very agitated, Alexis.'

*

I remember the first time I met HCA Robin. Robin had recently experienced her own loss of a relative. I found her warm, friendly, and non-judgemental. On my first day in Primrose, she said, 'Come with me, Alexis. Let's have a chat. How are you finding it here?'

I said, 'Well, it's fucking shit, isn't it?'

I spent a lot of time with Robin. She was one of the few staff who bothered to get to know me. Robin made time when there didn't seem to be any. HCAs like her are the unsung and poorly paid heroes of the NHS.

I should mention that before I was in hospital, my language was quite different. It changed as I learnt to survive.

At this stage nothing untoward had happened to me. I had about a week before things quickly escalated. I could feel something building. I was keeping a lot inside. I wasn't sure what it was. I didn't get the chance to pinpoint or talk it through. "It", whatever it was, felt stuck inside, something I didn't understand and wasn't able to express.

From the staff's perspective, one minute everything was fine and the next I was out of control. I was like a balloon that had been pumped up too much. The ward was a place where no air could escape the balloon, so even the faintest puff of breath could cause an outburst. The staff's answer to this was to keep me sedated. My mum said I was like a zombie. I was on methylphenidate, escitalopram, quetiapine, zopiclone, promethazine, and diazepam. It was the beginning of polypharmacy and addiction.

After two weeks of this, I felt extremely ill. I had lost everything. I lost my home in Asia because I had moved. These medical people would say, 'Oh, so you live with your parents?' Yeah, I currently live with my parents, but I've been living independently since I was aged 15.

They would say, 'Oh, so you self-harm?' It was very embarrassing and degrading. They take all your stuff away from you, even your belt. I was very much into fitness but I couldn't even have my skipping rope. You lose your identity. You become this sick thing. Then you think, *I am really ill.*

Mental distress has no bedtime. Throughout the night, noise seeped through the walls. The sounds of people shouting, screaming, and pacing entered my room and my dreams. Alarms would go off even in the night time if somebody kicked off.

It's hard to sleep on a psych ward. Every room door has a small window. The window is made with slats that slide to reveal strips of about one centimetre of space to see through. Although you can open the window or close it, staff have ultimate control from the outside. Regardless of the observation you're on, 10-minute, 15-minute, 30-minute or hourly, they open the slats and shine a torch at you. They shine it until they know you are safe and well. At night it's usually until they can see your chest rising and falling. This may take a while if you're in a position where your chest is covered. I couldn't sleep because I was so sensitive to the torch light and the noise.

CHAPTER 9

Occupational Therapy

During the day, we had an occupational therapist, but she was actually a glorified activities coordinator and bad at it. Her name was Kathy. She was mid-40s, with long, flowing brown hair and she wore spectacles. I found her to be quite fake, a puzzling lady. I could never work out whether she was well intentioned or not. Often, she would talk to me and be helpful. At other times, she seemed to suggest that I was bad, wrong, and a ticking time bomb capable of committing some horrific act.

Kathy didn't appreciate my expressions of individuality or preference for choice either. I remember when I used to express my feelings on the activities she offered, she would shut me down saying that I was monopolising. Really, I think she just didn't like me suggesting something that wasn't in keeping with the status quo.

A psychiatric ward is a structured place. I liked this. Kathy was a major part of its structure. So, she was important to me whether or not she was an easy person or what she offered was worthwhile. Everything in the ward was organised around food and medication. These were the only actions that were guaranteed to take place at roughly the same times. It was also the only time where both nurses and HCAs were on the floor.

The ward daily schedule was like this: You were awakened at seven o'clock. Due to meds and people's moods, most people fell out of bed an hour later. At eight o'clock, you had breakfast and got your medication. I didn't like breakfast because I have a phobia of fruit. I've had this problem since I was born. The smell, taste, and texture are too strong for me. Also, the non-existent table manners bothered me so I tried to eat early when nobody was around.

When it was time for medication, everyone had to line up. I hated that. Most people didn't want the drugs, yet you had to line up for them. And everyone could hear what you were having. Then there was the security thing. There was a hatch and you had to get the medication from there. The hatch looked like a horse stable with the nurse in the stable part, protected from us patients by a barrier.

Then at 9.30am, there was a morning meeting where we discussed what activities we wanted to do on the ward. And there was daily news. This group was called "Morning Meeting and Current Affairs". Those of us that turned up would each be given a piece of paper. I went there because it was something to do to take my mind off things. The paper contained a news story. But it wasn't the real news. Never mind that the Brits and Americans are bombing Iraq. It would be like a cat got stuck up a tree and a fireman got it down. Or they've made a robot in Japan that can make tea. It was patronising. I didn't care whether a robot could make a cup of tea.

Drinks were another challenge. There was a tap you could push which dispensed either very cold water or lukewarm water for "hot drinks". The cups were plastic mugs. During the summer, ants would crawl over the drinks station because of the sugar. The tea and coffee were disgusting as the water was never hot enough to dissolve the granules or brew the tea. And you were only allowed this privilege at certain times of day. At random times, and stocks permitting, there were biscuits. A member of staff would put them out for us. We would swarm the drinks station to get them like a pack of animals chewing up a fresh kill. When I first saw this happen, I looked on in horror. After a while I was one of the pack.

Before lunch, at ten o'clock, there would be a group activity, like bracelet making where you plait yarn or beads. Surprisingly, even the men joined in too.

You had your second meds at twelve o'clock. Lunch was at 12.30pm. The whole lunch situation was the same as breakfast for me. And I couldn't put food in my mouth anyway. It was too heavy and the taste was too strong.

Then in the afternoon there would be a group activity from two o'clock to three o'clock, like papier-mâché or something like that.

After that, from three o'clock till four o'clock, if you had leave you could go off the ward with the OT once a week on a Wednesday. You could go into the community to walk to the shop. But I rarely had that leave. Even when I had leave, it seemed as though Kathy would find a reason not to take me. Then at five o'clock, there were more meds, served alongside dinner.

That was it.

Visiting hours were the hour before dinner and meds, from four o'clock until five o'clock, and then after dinner for two hours from six o'clock until eight o'clock. At these times, you could see how marginalised so-called mental patients were. Only about a third of the ward was visited regularly. Some people were never visited. To start with, I had quite a few visitors. As time progressed the numbers dwindled to less than a handful. My mum would come as much as she could. My dad never came because he was always in conflict with the managers. He didn't agree with what they were doing and how I was treated. I could count the number of times Thomas came on one hand.

My biggest problem was not being able to see Abi. She was the person I most wanted. Because she was less than a year old, she would be sleeping during visiting hours. I also didn't want her on a ward. I relied a lot on getting leave off the ward. When I did visit her off the ward and then had to go back, I felt like the worst parent. The whole visiting situation was difficult for everybody. I felt isolated when no visitors showed up.

Wednesday was my favourite day, because in the afternoon there was a fitness class. It was doleful, but at least I was moving. There were two options: a sitting-in-a-chair fitness option and a regular stand-up-and-move option. The leader of the class, Ariana, was nice. She was about 60 years old and very fit. I think she had experienced extreme emotional distress so she had more compassion than some of the other staff. She made a third option for me and pushed me hard. I felt much better after taking her group. She would always talk to me afterwards. I felt like she saw me as a person, not a monster.

Art therapy was in the morning. The first week I was in Primrose Ward, the art therapist, Julia, would say, 'You know, Alexis, you should come to art therapy.' She had been doing it for 30 years. She retired from work when I was still in the unit.

I said, 'I hate drawing. Just go away from me. Don't speak to me. You're hurting my ears.'

The next week she said, 'Come, Alexis. Come to art therapy.'

I said, 'I can't draw.'

The next week she came over to me. I said, 'Look, I'm not coming, Julia. Just leave me alone, please.'

On the fourth week I gave in and said, 'Okay, I'm going.' So, I went there and never stopped drawing after that. She was a very difficult lady, Julia, very old-fashioned.

Every session, she would say the same thing, and I found that comforting. At the start of class, she would say, 'Just take your pencil for a walk along the paper and see what you can create.' I loved the repetitive nature of her few words. It was because of Julia that I became able to express myself. Then I was drawing all the time.

But there was an incident in the art room. I had a paintbrush. I wiped the paintbrush with tissue paper to get the paint off. I went to the bin, the kind where you put your foot on the lever at the bottom and the lid opens. I put the paper inside. I was struggling to understand how much pressure you need to apply to things. I had lost that ability to understand how much force things needed to work. The bin lid was metal and shut loudly with a BANG. Julia said, 'Alexis, why are you doing that? That's very rude. You are disrupting the group.'

I told her, 'Julia, I'm very sorry, but I'm not disrupting the group. I didn't mean to do that. It was an accident.'

Then she said in a confrontational voice, 'What's wrong with you? What's wrong with you?'

I told her, 'There's nothing wrong with me, Julia. Just back off.' I sat down and she pressed the alarm, doot-doot-doot-doot. I was holding my ears.

They all came in, and I said, 'There's no problem here. Just back off. There's no problem here.'

But they told me, 'You need to leave, Alexis.'

I find it really hard to switch tasks, especially when I am stressed and I am expected to do it instantly. I said to them, 'I'm sorry, I can't leave because I haven't finished. I'm just changing the colour of my paint.'

'That's it for today, Alexis. You must go now.'

'I can't go because I have to finish this picture. I've only been here for 10 minutes, and the session is for 60 minutes, so you need to allow me to finish and I have a plan for the piece I am working on.'

'We're not allowing you to finish. You either move now or we will move you.'

'Well, I'm sorry. I can't move. Just let me finish.' Then they grabbed me by my arms. That was so much pain. They pulled me out and put me in the calming room. There's nothing calm about the calming room. You go into the calming room when you're not calm. They pushed me onto the floor. At least it's a little bit padded in there, like a running track. Then they injected me. After that I didn't like to go to art because I was too worried that I would make a mistake. But I kept drawing.

*

I complained about the art room incident. I received a signed letter from the CEO. It stated:

... you resisted nursing staff instructions, you were ultimately restrained.

While acknowledging that your behaviour disrupted the other patients she (the investigator) *does not feel that everything was done to de-escalate the situation and avoid restraint. The important of de-escalation is emphasised in training as restraint is emotionally traumatic for patients ...*

I apologise for the apparent distress this caused.

CHAPTER 10

Meltdown

A meltdown differs from what's called "kicking off". Kicking off comes out of frustration or anger, or a need to escape. There's usually a goal in mind, like getting away or needing something attended to. And there's some ability to control the physical behaviour. Meltdowns, however, are beyond anyone's control.

My head would have a very strange feeling, like the balloon I described exploding, right before it happened. Pressure builds and pushes on my skull from the inside out. I can't think or talk because it hurts. I can only shout or scream.

Moving was good. For me it was mostly pacing back and forth. I wanted to hit something or push against the wall, but mostly I avoided this for fear of harming myself or looking crazy. Yet it helped me to know where I was in space and time. Nobody knew why this was happening. I would run up and down the corridors to try to get rid of the feeling.

I was filled to the bursting point with the noise, the smell, and all these new people. Some emotions were months old and unexpressed. I was thinking back to my move, my old job, the birth of Abi, the longing to sit on a wave in the ocean and ride it in. That freedom was all gone. This flitted around my brain, unable to emerge in any coherent way. The pressure just burst out of me. If they had only listened, like HCA Robin did. But they did not listen to me, or to her.

Robin would say, 'Alexis needs to go out. Let me take her out.'

They would say, 'No, she is not going out.'

Robin would tell me, 'Lexi, you need to calm down, be quiet for a few days, and they'll let you out. Stay in your room, go in the courtyard, try to stay settled, and they'll let you go.' But it just got worse and worse until the restraints started.

I have been restrained 96 times in the NHS. I learnt this from my NHS records. Most of these were in response to not "reining it in" and for not controlling how I expressed myself to make sense to anyone. So, when I went into meltdown, usually an HCA would come, because the nurses were too busy. The nurses rarely came out of their bloody glass office. The HCAs would talk – they were on the floor.

I couldn't process the information they were communicating. It was like a visual and auditory assault on my brain. This made everything worse.

I would get so frustrated that I couldn't speak. They would scold me: 'You need to answer me, Alexis. Why aren't you answering me? You're capable of answering me, Alexis. You need to listen, and you need to answer me.' Talking at me really wasn't helpful. When I couldn't respond in a way they understood, they took action.

Remember that I am 6'1" and very athletic. Someone would push an alarm on their belt. This started the high-pitched **doot-doot-doot-doot** sound. At least four people, maybe six, would come. Three from the ward I was on, three from other units in the hospital. This was a standard procedure. The staff would immobilise me by taking over my movement in a standing, sitting or prone position, depending on where I was, what I was doing, and where was easiest for them. They would smash me onto the floor. One might hold my head down onto the floor. For the first two years it was always a face-down restraint.

One would be on each arm, pressing them straight out like a starfish. They would lean in to my body. There was also one on each leg, and one just talking at me. This was how they controlled me, and by injection too – a chemical restraint.

One of these times, a nurse very calmly left the restraint and walked fast to the clinical room. She came out with a cardboard kidney tray with a paper towel on top covering the contents. Then I saw the syringe. In front of everyone the staff pulled down my pants. A nurse administered the injection aggressively, like a stab.

All of their grabbing felt like fire. It started off like pins and needles, then became burning. I would try to get them off. I felt pinned and helpless and not fully aware.

They injected me with benzodiazepine, sometimes mixed with something else like promethazine or olanzapine. Then I would sleep for a few hours. Because I had slept they thought their treatment was helping – the system calls this "responding to medication with good effect".

This was where the whole compliance thing started. If you don't do exactly what they say, when they say, you're in trouble. They hold all the power and they own you. They can restrain you when they like and fill you with chemicals when they like. That's why Robin kept telling me, 'Just do what they ask, Lexi, and you'll be fine.'

But I wasn't fine. I was now addicted to some of the drugs and I craved them. They increased the dosages because I was developing a tolerance. And now when I got the jabs, they were giving me two drugs, which acted like a cosh. When I told them, 'This isn't good. I'm just getting worse,' they told me I was "lacking insight into my condition".

At this time, in January and February, my mum and dad could see a huge deterioration in me. I just thought there was something terribly wrong. I'd never been like this before. What is this all about? I couldn't understand it.

I became more desperately sad. My life was exhausting. What I struggled with, everyone thought was minor. Nothing that was intolerable to me seemed to bother or annoy anyone else. My responses were extreme agitation or anger that was totally unacceptable by the ward.

They decided rather too quickly for my liking that I had Emotionally Unstable Personality Disorder (EUPD). What? My personality is disordered? Since when? Despite taking the drugs and accepting treatment, I got worse and worse. It seemed their medical interventions had the opposite effect they were designed for. My parents said, 'She absolutely does not have that,' and were fighting the diagnosis. EUPD was my primary diagnosis for the next year and a half. I was acting out, I don't deny it. The professionals thought I was doing it for attention, being manipulative or something. This change in me had all happened in a month. My personality was never considered "disordered" before.

CHAPTER 11

Ruby

A patient named Ruby was bullying me. She kept saying I was weird, being nasty to me, taking the mickey out of me because I would respond slowly. She made fun of my voice, called me a man, or said my daughter was an "N-word" because she's mixed-race – my ex-partner being Nigerian. The staff didn't intervene. This went on for days. It was not like I could stay away from her, because there was nowhere to go.

Finally, I shouted at her, 'How dare you speak to me like that. Even if you are ill, you need to have respect for other people.'

Then the staff came. I told them, 'This is racism. This is abusive harassment. If you don't stop this, I will call the police.'

So, they moved her to the other ward, but it was joined to my ward. She used to come up to the door and smack it, shouting, 'Alexis,' and abuse through the door.

I said to the staff, 'She needs to move somewhere else. Even when she's in a different ward she's still abusing me. You're not doing anything about it.' They stuck paper to the door so I couldn't see her.

In that week I was assaulted twice more. Once I was in the meds room with a male patient who groped me in front of a female nurse. She asked him to stop. Another day I was sitting at a table and a female patient pounded me with her fists, a volley of rolling punches to my face. Each time, my meltdown response got me drugged or restrained.

The CEO of the Trust replied to my complaint:

It is regrettable that these incidents occurred and it is apparent that they were very distressing. It is unfortunate incidents like this occur due to the acute nature of the patients admitted.

They had no compassion. I continued to live in fear.

As I had more meltdowns, everyone with any medical training would tell me, 'Alexis, you are very sick. You are very unstable. You have to take this medication.' My dose of benzos increased. I was being treated because my brain was ill. So many things were not right, even my eating.

'Why don't you eat?' They challenged me, like I was not eating on purpose. But I couldn't do it. I could do nothing. I was trying my best and it was no way near good enough. Robin spent time trying to understand, but that was all.

Eventually I was sectioned. Apparently, I was a danger to myself from the self-harm and meltdowns. They put me on obs. Now I not only had the sensory overload of the physical environment, but I also had two people invading my space, watching me at all times.

The observers rarely want to interact with you. The good ones will, though. They might play Scrabble or Connect 4 or similar games. However, mostly staff feel like you are a waste of time because you don't have a "true" mental illness like schizophrenia or bipolar. My "condition" was not "organic" and therefore I was acting out – like a child. Staff watch you every minute of the day and make it known that your behaviour is wilful and a waste of NHS resources.

The obs are invasive. If you go to the toilet, they watch you. Even if you say to them, 'I need to get changed. Can you look the other way, please?', they won't. They don't let you shower or bathe on your own. So, you don't want to shower or go to the toilet because it's embarrassing. Then you can get constipated. You can get a bad stomach ache and sick. Sometimes, if Robin was on, she would let me go to the toilet on my own. I would just tell her, 'I won't do anything, Robin. Please, can you just let me go on my own?'

As my reactions to situations worsened, I sought strategies to calm myself. I realised if I wrapped myself tightly in something, it was very comforting. So, I used to wrap a blanket around me. That deep pressure felt good. But this strategy didn't come without its problems. Sometimes when a nurse I didn't know was on shift they would think I was trying to suffocate myself so they didn't let me do it. Especially when on obs, this calming strategy was rarely permitted. When I was being observed I felt like a science experiment. They would medicate me and see what happened, put people watching me and see what happened. But nothing positive happened. Things just got worse.

CHAPTER 12

Unique Diagnosis

There's something addictive about self-harm. For me it gave a sense of predictability when nothing was predictable. When I was doing it, I was like, *What is that? What just happened?* I didn't know why I was cutting, yet the need to do it was strong.

I was desperate. One day I got a blade. I went into the clinic room for a daily blood pressure check. I saw the sharps box there. A sharps box is a hard plastic container used to safely dispose of hypodermic needles and other sharp medical instruments, such as IV catheters and disposable scalpels.

Because I'd been on obs, I hadn't been able to cut. I went to the box and took a "sharp" from there. It's hard to believe that I was in such a desperate state that I took a used "sharp" and cut my arm. I didn't know what was happening. I couldn't get out of this transfixed mindset. It was as if I wasn't in myself.

Craig was there, the deputy ward manager. He was about 5'8" with a bald head. He looked like a judo player. Craig was slender, muscular, and toned. He just wrestled me onto the ground and pressed the alarm – **doot-doot-doot-doot**. Everyone came running. They all jumped on me. I wasn't inside my mind. I was watching from the outside.

I couldn't follow their instructions because I couldn't make sense of what they were saying. All the sensory signals were mixed up – light, sound, smell, pressure were not making sense in my mind. For lots of reasons I found I couldn't let go of the blade.

I was on the floor, all spread-eagled during the restraint by six staff. Craig grabbed the blade with his gloves. Some staff wore blue gloves. It was the procedure for restraint and injections. Craig exclaimed, 'You fucking bitch, Alexis.' I couldn't respond to ask him why I was a fucking bitch. Later I learnt that where he had taken the blade, it had cut through his gloves. Fortunately, it didn't break his skin. I felt bad after. I liked Craig. He was a very candid guy. He cared a lot about his job.

Later, I was in my room on obs, and Craig said, 'You know, Alexis, what your problem is? You have "Fucking Bitch Disorder".' It was times like this where I felt bad, but I was also fuming with them. I hated myself and what I had become. Staff could be very cruel sometimes.

CHAPTER 13

Nurse Logan

I had nightmares about stuff that had happened, mostly restraints. Once I woke up from a nightmare at two o'clock in the morning. By this time, I was addicted to diazepam, a benzodiazepine. So I asked the agency staff named Logan, 'Excuse me, please can I talk to the nurse? I need to have some PRN lorazepam.' PRN is an abbreviation meaning "as needed" medication from the Latin *pro re nata,* for an occasion that has arisen, or as circumstances require it.

He told me, 'The nurse isn't available tonight.'

HCA Robin was also on shift so I waited for an hour, and then said to her, 'I need to have some PRN lorazepam. I can't sleep because I keep having the same nightmare.' Every time I closed my eyes, it was very vivid. It's not that I was seeing what had happened. It was like I was back in that very moment. I'd wake up struggling to breathe, gasping for air with my heart racing and a sick feeling in my stomach.

She told me, 'That is the nurse, Alexis. You were talking to him an hour ago.'

'Logan? He told me he's not the nurse, that there was no nurse on shift. He just lied.'

So, I asked Nurse Logan, 'Why did you lie to me?'

He said, 'Oh, I didn't have time to get your PRN medication.'

Then I had a meltdown. 'Why didn't you just say "I'm a bit busy, can you come back in 10 minutes," instead of telling me there's no nurse on duty?' I shouted. Doot-doot-doot, he set the alarm off. I panicked and ran. Not that there was anywhere to run.

Restraint followed.

CHAPTER 14

Maisie and Compassion or Lack Of

There was a girl in Primrose Ward called Maisie. She was experiencing extreme states of emotion and they were going to discharge her. She didn't want that. She punched the wall in anger and broke her hand. Her discharge was in a few days, because they had to find a bedsit for her. Maisie was effectively homeless. Now she had a broken hand, and they wouldn't help her to the hospital to cast it. She didn't know where the hospital was. She was in so much pain she was crying.

I knew the area quite well. Although I didn't identify with her crying, I knew she needed to get the hand cast. All they had thought to do was to roll up a magazine around her arm and tie it together, which is not the way at all to deal with a break. It would've been better to just leave it alone. They said they were going to give treatment, but they didn't have staff so they couldn't do anything until the next day when the new shift came on.

I said to Maisie, 'Come on, let's go.' We walked to the hospital, which was 3.3 kilometres away. It took about an hour to get there.

Maisie's hand was broken in two places. She had a cast put on, and by the time everything was done it was eleven o'clock at night. Because we were psychiatric patients, they had taken us in faster. They didn't like us hanging around. That was a benefit to being us, I guessed.

I don't respond well in a hospital, so I was stimming and pacing. I have quite a lot of self-stimulating behaviours when experiencing sensory overload or high levels of anxiety, for example, repetitive motion such as bouncing my knees, flicking my fingers, repeating numbers, and repetitive movement of objects. More well-known stims among the autistic community are hand flapping and rocking. Stimming feels good to me and counteracted the busy, chaotic sensory environment of the hospital. However, some people find stimming disturbing and make this known.

*

I called the psych ward after we were done. It was dark, in the middle of Heysham, we had no money, and it was raining. They said they would not pick us up. So, I phoned my mum, and said, 'This is really bad. It's dangerous. Can you come get us?'

She said, 'Lexi, I'm 40 minutes away in Morecombe Cove.' I sent her the picture of Maisie's arm in the magazine, and in the splint. She was fuming, so she phoned the hospital up. They sent a taxi to get us.

The next day I got such an ear-bashing from the consultant. 'You shouldn't be interfering. This had nothing to do with you.' They complained that I was aloof and antisocial and then when I helped somebody, they complained about that too.

That's the thing, though. It is to do with me. You meet these people and you don't want to see anyone in unnecessary pain. They were going to leave her like that all night, all night with no treatment. It's unacceptable. It's more than a lack of compassion. It's not humane. And when you can do something so easily, just show her where the hospital is, take her there and sit with her, why would you not do that?

The attitude of the physical health staff in the hospital leaves a lot to be desired. They often say to those of us who self-harm, 'Well, it's your own fault. You did that to yourself.' Maisie was no different. She got the same speech. Obviously, she broke her arm for attention (sarcasm intended).

I remember one time I had cut myself. To go to hospital, the doctor has to come, assess you, and agree you need to go. Otherwise you can't leave the unit. So, the doctor came to see me, and said, 'You need to have stitches, but you can't go for a few hours.'

'Well, that's really not helpful, is it?'

'It's really not helpful that you cut yourself on purpose and drain NHS money.'

Like I wanted to be sectioned, have my liberty denied, be humiliated, or get more and more addicted to drugs that weren't helping. Nobody would want to live the way I was living. Their judgement-laden attitude was incredible. This was what physical health doctors felt about self-harmers. I think they get a lot of their attitude from psychiatry.

I learnt that mental health doctors call people diagnosed with personality disorder "Dracula". Why? Because we suck all the life and resources out of the service with our so-called "illness". It's still largely considered a social disorder without a biological basis.

Another time when I went to hospital to get stitched up, the doctor said, 'You know, I never wanted to go into psychiatry. It's a complete waste of time. There's no way any of you guys are going to get better.' He thought that was a fine way to talk. But who can blame him when his colleagues over in the psych ward are calling us Dracula! The hope narrative is sadly lacking.

CHAPTER 15

Leg Injury

When you are in pain, desperate, and you know no other way to cope, cutting becomes a learnt option. I can see how from staff's perspective it was concerning. But it was not about dying at this point. It was the drug. The cutting had never been prolific, but it was getting bolder every time.

I was on 1:1 obs with a young HCA named Ava. We were in the art room and I asked for the pencil sharpener. I was drawing a lot then because I couldn't express myself verbally. I started sharpening the pencil. I don't know what changed in my mind but what followed seemed to just happen. I smashed the pencil sharpener and went for my neck. Ava jumped on my back. She pushed my hands down, so all I could get to was my leg. I hadn't set out to make the huge incision that followed, or any incision. Because she was pressing on me, and I was feeling fire all over I cut my leg – twice. That was the worst self-injury I have ever made. I have two long scars on my leg from my knee almost to my groin. I had 47 stitches in one cut.

To give you an idea of the extent of my self-harm, I have 26 scars that I inflicted on myself.

I hated what I was doing to myself.

CHAPTER 16

Care Programme Approach Meeting

By law, every six months you must have a CPA (Care Programme Approach) meeting to plan your treatment. I wasn't getting any treatment. A sizeable proportion of people in acute units are not there for treatment. They are in for containment until staff can find somewhere else for them to go. Maybe some people with acute psychosis are treated with medication and maybe they get better. But generally, it's a holding ground. Either people are homeless or suffering addiction and are being held until there is a place for them to live, or people like me and especially people labelled with severe personality disorders – there are always a couple in every unit – are being held until funding is available to move them. So, with a bed crisis, it can take nine months to a year, maybe even several years, for funding to be approved.

You have these CPA meetings, which in my experience were a tick-box exercise, nothing about care. They always concluded with 'do more of the same' – drug treatment and firefighting. In acute they're every four to six weeks.

My mum and dad were at the Primrose meeting, and they were strong. They asked, 'What are you actually doing to help Alexis? She came to you as a professional woman in crisis distressed state, and now she can hardly function. What treatment are you providing for her?'

I'd been in Primrose Ward for 10 weeks, and my mum and dad had phoned repeatedly because they wanted to talk about the quetiapine. Dr Dempsey, the responsible clinician (RC), kept ignoring their calls. They complained to what's called the Patient Experience Team who manages complaints. They got no response at first.

Eventually Dr Dempsey makes herself available. After five minutes of my mum explaining why she wanted to talk about this medication, the doctor started looking at her watch. We let it go a few times. The clock was behind her on the wall. I said, 'Just so you know, Dr Dempsey, it's 3.07pm, if that's helpful.'

'Oh, you know, Alexis, I just don't have time to talk at this length. I don't have time.'

My mum says to her, 'You haven't had time for 10 weeks. We really need to discuss this medication with you. Why haven't you replied to my phone calls or any of my letters?'

'I just don't have time to deal with this situation.'

My mother says, 'What? In 10 weeks?'

So that's how it is. They just didn't give a shit. Or that was how it felt. To give a shit, they would have needed double the resources, half the workload, work with a theory of mental health beyond the medical model, gain a bucket load of understanding and some compassion – but they had none of that. In the end Dr Dempsey prescribed the same treatment. The quetiapine wasn't stopped. They wrote:

You say that you have made it firmly known to Dr Dempsey that you are concerned about this drug, and the adverse effects it may have on Alexis. Please be advised that as the Consultant responsible for Alexis's care and treatment, she is qualified and experienced in the use of psychotropic medication and is aware of the benefits and risks associated with such treatments.

CHAPTER 17

Cage Transfer

After the accident with my leg, I was on obs. I wanted to go to sleep and never wake up.

One night while I was sleeping, suddenly my eyes were flooded with light. Six figures surrounded my bed. It took a while to realise I wasn't dreaming. A figure spoke. It was Paola, the small European nurse and deputy ward manager. She was called the Poisonous Dwarf by her own staff. Paola was heartless and matter of fact in her approach, in an underhand way. You never knew what to expect from her. Now she was direct, cold, and sure of herself. She had an agenda.

The time was 1.37am. Groggily, I asked, 'What the fuck's going on?'

Paola said, 'You are being transferred.'

This was the first time I'd been transferred. I asked, 'Transferred to where?'

'You're going to a different hospital, leaving Blackthorn,' Paola said.

I said, 'Right. Well, I don't want to go, thanks.' As I looked around my room, I saw all my stuff had been packed. The wardrobe and open shelves were cleaned out. Everything was gone. They had done it while I was heavily sedated. Since I wore earplugs and ear defenders, I hadn't heard a single thing. I felt suddenly invaded and under threat. My heart was beating hard and I had trouble breathing.

I hated it at Primrose, but I hated change more. And they hadn't even told me so I could prepare! I didn't know where I was going. I didn't want to leave my daughter and my family. I told them again I wasn't going. I asked them to let me sleep, and could we discuss it in the morning.

Then they all grabbed me. I shouted and screamed. My skin was on fire. The room was suddenly far too bright. The noise of the alarms was piercing my ears. I was resisting. I had to get free. Now my brain was exploding.

I was dragged along the corridor. They pulled down my trousers and underpants. With my bare bottom exposed, I felt the needle pierce my skin. A nurse grabbed the waistline of my trousers and held me by it. I could feel their hot, sweaty hands on my bum. Then I was outside. The fresh air was cooling. I saw the ambulance. But I wasn't sick.

I wasn't sick.

I was looking at it from the floor where my head was turned to the side, pressed onto the floor by staff. As I struggled to breathe, I saw the ambulance doors open. This was no ordinary ambulance. Inside, there was a cage. My eyes squinted against the impossibility of what I saw. This was like the cages dogs are impounded in. I was fuming. A wave of heat overtook me as I worked out that they actually wanted to put me in the cage. Like a dog, like an animal. I screamed out, 'I'm not getting in there.'

Soon the drug brought calmness. Sedated, I didn't have the energy to fight, but inside I felt shock, trauma, hopelessness. I conceded, but said, 'I'll just sit inside the car. I'll go, but I don't want to sit in a cage.' A last-ditch effort at humanity was worth a try.

They said, 'No. You have to sit in the cage. You're being transferred.' I tried not to get inside the cage.

They got me in. They locked the door and put a bright light on inside. It was a lightning bolt through my eyes. It was like the light you see in an operating theatre, reflecting off the cream-coloured walls inside the ambulance. As I tried to adjust to my new reality, the cage rattled and squeaked with every bump in the road. The journey was long, about an hour.

I felt like I had just been violated physically, mentally, and emotionally. What had just happened? Usually a person who enters your sleeping space at night, takes your stuff without your permission, assaults you, pulls down your pants needs to act discreetly. They rightly fear criminal charges.

Such perpetrators rarely get to carry out their assault on a victim with the enthusiastic participation of half a dozen buddies in a government building masquerading as a hospital.

How absurd. In those moments when I regained my mind, I wanted to call the police. However, I knew the criminal justice system wouldn't be interested. Unlike a regular human, my situation was different. My perpetrators wouldn't be arrested for their acts. Instead they would receive a favourable reaction as they justify themselves under the pretence that I lacked receptivity caused by a "chemical imbalance". I was ill and was being unreasonable in my behavioural resistance, because, as everyone knows, non-compliance is mediated by neurotransmitters and hormones.

I asked the staff in the back of the transport, 'Can I speak to my mum to tell her I'm being transferred?' They wouldn't allow that. So, I just sat there in the cage with my brain full. I was overwhelmed by what I guessed was emotion. I was sitting in a cage. I was in a cage. I would like to tell you I cried. I did my own version of crying which to an observer looked like nothing. I just sat in their cage and looked at the bars because there was nothing else to look at. I counted the squares instead of lamp posts. This was the best I could do to keep calm.

I didn't want to go inside the ward, because I didn't know what was coming. When the ambulance door opened, I tried to stay in the cage. When they got me out, I tried hard not to go through the first door to the hospital. I breathed in the cold, crisp winter air, knowing I wouldn't see this side of the hospital for a long time. When they got me through the first door, I oriented myself to the foyer. I did my best to stay there. There were three more doors to ward confinement hell. Then I was in the airlock. There's a door and a big space, maybe 10 metres, and another door. You can't run through the doors. You wouldn't make it because both doors don't open at the same time.

They did this to me two more times, always to a psychiatric intensive care unit, a PICU. These are for people considered to be in an acutely disturbed state of mental disorder. Each time it happened at midnight when they knew I would be asleep. Staff packed by stealth and surprised me. After the first time, I asked them not to do it again, but that did no good.

CHAPTER 18

Seclusion

They had dragged me along a 30-metre corridor and into a white room with a rubber type floor. I recognised the same NHS-issue blue mattress in there. I didn't know where I was, but because of the mattress at least I knew it was an NHS facility. This was my first experience of seclusion.

Staff force you onto the mattress face down. Your head faces the wall and your feet face the door. They press your arms down, one person on each, then they cross your legs and bend your knees so your ankles touch your bum. They push your feet to your bum with your legs crossed. It hurts a lot. It's hard to breathe, too, because the mattress is soft and you get embedded in it. My body wasn't made to contort in the ways they forced it.

After the injections, staff leave the room like a rehearsed military drill. This is called Promoting Safe and Therapeutic Services, or PSTS. The two people holding your feet leave first. Then the next two holding the legs follow. Then the next two who held your arms leave. The last one, on your head, runs out. Then you are alone. It takes about 20 minutes for the drugs to sedate you.

After a few hours I asked to use the toilet. There's no toilet, just four walls. Staff didn't respond. So, I had to urinate and defecate on the floor. This was probably one of the most degrading things I've done in my life. I am not shy to pee on the ground when I'm in the wilderness, jungle, or on the beach. Anyone who has been in Asia will know that you can't be precious about toilet facilities. But relieving yourself on the floor in a hospital with staff watching you, when you know there are perfectly good facilities just outside the room, is entirely different. It took me to a new low.

Every two hours, staff come to assess you. First, they knock on the window. If you've moved the mattress, they tell you to move it back into the corner of the room furthest from the door. Then you must sit next to the wall on the mattress with your legs straight. One member of staff comes in, and there are five or six people at the door. You know if you get up they're going after you. I've never tried to get up.

They ask, 'Alexis, can I give you an injection?' Obviously, you don't want one, but to say you don't is a bad idea.

After, you feel nothing. All your senses are completely dulled, you don't feel much. Sleep is welcome when you're in such a bad way.

Sitting in the room alone you get attuned to yourself. It's a heightened awareness of sounds, time, feelings of loss of control, and the awful thoughts I have thinking back over the midnight wake-up, and the reason I was sent to this place. Thinking what I was and what I've become. Sitting next to shit and pee and wondering why I am not good enough to use a damn toilet!

There were some things I liked about the seclusion room. The air-con unit was my favourite feature. It purred like a cat. Seclusion introduced me to the power of white noise. It was the only quiet, private place on the PICU so when I was overstimulated, it helped a bit. But the therapeutic benefit ends with the air con.

It's much quicker and easier to lock somebody in a room than to talk things through, identify triggers in the environment, and make adjustments. I have been secluded 17 times. Seclusion is a constant threat of extreme punishment hanging over your head. It's wrong. There's nothing therapeutic about the force that comes with the act. The aggressive removal of my clothes, other belongings, and the forceful injection of medications is inhumane. I was powerless. Sometimes the quiet time had the benefit that I regained control of myself. But there are many better ways to help someone than to lock them in a room. After a while sensory deprivation loses its calming effect. You focus on the fact that you can't do a thing about the situation. Afterwards, no one would talk about what happened. I could have used a chat to work on how to avoid overload and meltdown, always the main reason for seclusion. These opportunities were as rare as a solar eclipse.

CHAPTER 19

PICU Ivy Suite

22nd May 2013

I was sent to Ivy Suite because of the leg cut. I thought, *Fine. I need intensive care. I am faulty. I am wrong. I am disordered.* My self-esteem was in the toilet.

Ivy Suite had its own entrance separate from the other units. Ambulances pulled up and got direct access to the ward. People didn't want to go in there, so you could hardly expect them to willingly walk through six doors! Once inside, there was no access to the outside world. Even the garden courtyard was inside the hospital. As a nature lover, I used to lie on the slabs in the middle of the courtyard, look at the sky and watch birds. There were no trees, just birds, and I would think, *God, I wish I could just fly away and be in the quiet with the wind.*

The best thing about PICU for me was the regular courtyard times. They would open the door exactly on the hour, and call everyone in exactly when time was up. The schedule on the door never changed. When I first went to PICU, smoking was still permitted in hospitals. Staff would shout, 'smoking time, smoking time'. People lined up for tobacco, and smoked cigarette after cigarette, to cope. After smoking was banned, staff would shout, 'fresh air, fresh air'.

The tables and chairs weren't bolted to the floor in this PICU dining area. There were occasions where patients would throw them – it was rare. All staff would flank the tables. We ate in the middle and staff stood in a circle around us. If anyone raised their voice, or there was any conflict, staff would be straight on it.

PICU was orderly. We were called by room number – although this was only for the first time I was there – the other times you were called by name in room number order. This was to make getting food fair and orderly. At lunch, the server in the hatch where you picked up food would shout, 'Room 1'. Only then could the Room 1 person stand up and get their plate. When that person sat down, they would call 'Room 2'. If you stood up at the wrong time, you'd get in trouble. You weren't given metal cutlery when you first arrived. You had to prove you weren't violent and going to attack someone with a knife. I didn't get metal straight away.

There were 12 rooms in Ivy Suite PICU. In the evening at dinner, staff called people from Room 12 to Room 1 to make it fair. People get irate about food so this system was good. One side effect of the antipsychotic olanzapine is hunger for carbs. By dinnertime, patients were starving. Olanzapine is a central reason many people are overweight.

The bedrooms were on either side of the dining room. Bedrooms 9 to 12 were next to the seclusion room. People new to the ward were given one of those rooms. As you got closer and closer to discharge, you moved towards the main door. Rooms 1 and 2 were right next to the exit door. I couldn't wait to move away from the seclusion room. Every time I was asked to move closer, I felt good about myself. I felt closer to freedom. The rooms near seclusion were noisy. Sometimes people were in seclusion for eight hours; banging, banging, hammering on the door, constantly screaming and howling. If you were in rooms 9 to 12, you had to contend with that.

Everywhere else was public. The doors were always open; even bedroom doors. The only closed door was to the glass office where the nurses sat. The ward was open-plan with zero blind spots because the distressed people were genuinely unpredictable and often aggressive. People in PICU can't be managed on the acute unit. Conflicts and fights happened regularly.

In PICU, all the drugs made concentration hard for me. Still, I played Scrabble and Backgammon. The high staff ratio, 6 staff to 12 people, meant we got a lot of interaction and one-to-one time. Staff played games with me because the other patients were so doped up they had no motivation. I was very competitive and took the games seriously. My win rate was very high.

PICU had a Therapeutic Activity Unit, the TAU. Twice a day people would leave the main ward area, and go through an airlock to the art room, a meeting room for OT classes, and a big games hall that housed loads of sports stuff. Shyam, the deputy ward manager, would let me use it a lot. I loved it there. It doesn't sound like much but it was stimulation and activity that helped make things bearable. Shyam tried his best to get us an extra, third, session in the evenings as well.

In the one-to-one sessions with staff, I could run on the treadmill. I would turn the speed right up and run fast for my whole hour. If some of the Nigerian staff, who were invariably good at table tennis, were working, I played with them. The TAU was the highlight of my day.

*

The self-harming became progressively worse as my drug intake increased. Acute Services wouldn't remove quetiapine on the say-so of my parents. Because I was addicted, I didn't challenge it. My body needed it by this time. Eventually, in Ivy Suite, Dr Saty, the responsible clinician, or RC, the guy in charge, listened to my parents and said, 'Okay, we'll try stopping it and see how she responds.' Within two weeks of being off the drug, 90% of self-harming ended. Clearly it was drug-induced.

I made several positive therapeutic relationships on PICU. Shyam was my favourite nurse. He talked to me a lot. He was a man of small stature, but he commanded a lot of respect from everyone. He was half Indian and half Scottish. His grey hair was short but with a long rat-tail ponytail. Shyam listened to me. He saw when I was struggling and would help as much as he could.

Another unexpected therapeutic benefit was that Shyam helped me change my special interest. I could be honest with him. I told him I found the lack of potential suicide options difficult. He understood I wasn't going to kill myself. We had a discussion around methods. I complained to him, 'All the doors are slanted so you can't put rope on them to hang. The sinks have no plugs – no drowning. There are no ligature points.' A habit of mine was to immediately look for them when I went into a room. It was unsettling for me to see such an environment designed to prevent suicide. Shyam understood me.

When I felt hopeless, Shyam and another nurse named Achala would talk with me. Achala was Mauritian. She would say, 'It's up to you, Lexi,' and 'It's all in your hands.' I didn't feel like anything was in my control, but at least Achala wasn't a hope killer. PICU's job was to stabilise people, so they were always hopeful because they saw progress in every person. This positivity rubbed off on me even though I wasn't sure I could change my situation.

CHAPTER 20

Accuphase

I had a lot of meltdowns in PICU because the environment was harsh, volatile, and restrictive. Drugs were the answer. In PICU they use harder drugs. I'll never forget the first time I was "Accuphased". Anastasia, a Greek nurse, was a larger-than-life lady who wore the most incredible clothes. Every shift she sported high heels, always patterned with bright colours or prints, short skirts, and tight shirts. Anastasia came to my room one day. When she entered, I could see that she was not alone. There were staff waiting outside the door. She had the kidney dish with paper on top, an injection poking out from the side.

She said in her Greek accent, 'Alexis, I want to give you an injection.' I was confused as I hadn't done anything. The injection must have been planned.

I said to her, 'You know, Anastasia, when this happens normally, I've done something.'

She said, 'This is going to really help you, Lex.'

'I don't think I need any more help, thanks.'

'It's going to relax you. You're going to feel a lot better after.'

I could see the people outside, and knew if I refused they would come in and jab me anyway. So, I "agreed" to it. She pulled my pants down and did one injection. This was unusual because I usually had two. I asked her what it was. 'Accuphase,' she said as if she had just given me a glass of water and left with her entourage.

I waited for the sedation but there was no immediate effect. This was weird. For a few hours I was thinking, *Nothing's happening.* After about eight hours it started. It was like my head was in a cloud and I couldn't see out. My mouth dribbled saliva. I could hardly sit up in my bed. It was like nothing I'd had before. I slept for two or three days. I even messed in my bed, because I couldn't get up to go to the toilet. After about 36 hours, I got up and moved, but I couldn't think. I had that injection three more times. Every time after the first, I fought and pleaded not to have it because it was so horrible.

Section 17

Section 17 is the part of the Mental Health Act which allows the doctor to grant a detained person leave of absence from hospital. It is the only legal means by which I could leave the hospital site. If you don't have Section 17 and you leave, you are Absent Without Leave, AWOL. In PICU, you could earn up to 30 minutes of Section 17 leave per 24 hours. You could only go out when it was light in case you ran away. Leave was always escorted, and you had to remain arms-length from the staff escorting you.

Earning leave was quite a challenge. Firstly, you had to have been in PICU one week. Secondly, you had to be settled for 72 hours. Then you had to wait to see the doctor to write up the leave for you. Each patient sees the doctor only once a week, so it could be a matter of five or six days before leave was granted even though you'd been settled for the required time. Often, I would get to the 72 hours, then I might get overloaded, shout, or have a meltdown. I'd have to start all over again. My heart broke whenever this happened.

In an acute unit, you could get a lot of leave. It was during Section 17 I went home for the day to see Abi. In acute, when the doctor had written the leave paperwork and then an incident occurred, staff would pull you into the office and tear up the paperwork in front of your face. They never did that in PICU. They would say, 'Alexis, because of what's happened ...' But anyway, you knew that, because it was always the same for everyone. At least staff treated you with respect.

The 30 minutes of Section 17 leave seemed such a small thing but they meant the world to me. It was a time when you felt some normal freedom, and where you could call your loved ones. Inside PICU phones were not allowed so when I was out I used to catch up with my social media.

CHAPTER 22

Appalling

20th June 2013

This time, after three months in PICU, I became eligible for transfer back to acute services. Shyam told me I was being moved back to Clover Ward as this was the only bed available in the county. It was a horrible ward, but I was looking forward to more freedom and being closer to home.

My named nurse, Cynthia, drove me there. The named nurse is responsible for your case. They coordinate your care, write care plans, inform you of your rights and treatment options, liaise with family and help arrange transfer and discharge. Cynthia is quite an old, experienced nurse having worked at Ivy Suite PICU for many years. She is also kind and open-minded. Cynthia used to play a lot of backgammon with me. I was pleased she was with me for the transfer. It was a long drive and we chatted the entire way.

We travelled comfortably together in a taxi. It was pleasant sitting next to somebody on equal footing. In the taxi, Cynthia and I could have had any relationship; friends, mother and daughter, or colleagues. The taxi was normalising. Moving back to acute, I had been downgraded from low secure to an "open unit", so I didn't have to go in the cage. I enjoyed looking out the taxi window observing the outside world I hadn't seen for months.

When Cynthia and I arrived at Clover, staff greeted me, 'Oh, you're back again, Alexis. Let's see how long this lasts.' *Oh, good,* I thought, taking her comment literally. *Maybe this means I'll only be here a week.*

They took me to my room and left me. Cynthia didn't come with me but went to the glass office for the handover. This is where she handed over my medical notes, drugs card, and the stuff I wasn't allowed to keep like earphones, razors, belts, jewellery.

I put my bag down in my room and looked around. The room was dirty. The bed was unmade. It had the "just slept in" look, complete with a head-shaped indentation in the pillow. This triggered some explosive feeling inside me. I left the room fuming and said to staff, 'I've worked for three months to get out of PICU. I was looking forward to coming here, and you are rude to me on entry. Then you have the audacity to put me in a room you haven't even been bothered to clean.' Cynthia and my mum were there.

'Oh, for goodness sakes, Alexis, just go to your room.' They used to say that a lot. 'Just go to your room', like I was child. I did go. I got the duvet and brought it out.

'Look. Would you sleep in this? It's disgusting. There are hairs and stains on it.'

Cynthia said to the nurse, 'You need to do something about that.' The Clover nurse went with me.

The nurse said, 'The person in this room has just left. We'll change it tomorrow when the cleaners come.'

I was clear, 'No, no. We're not going to change it tomorrow. We're going to change it now.'

'Well, it's not my job.'

I said, 'Just give me the fucking cleaning stuff and I'll do it myself. I'm not sleeping in that. It's disgusting.' It was a weird feeling because I was cross with Clover staff, but relieved to be there and out of PICU. I couldn't wait for the freedom, the Section 17 leave, to see my family and be closer to home.

This is what my life was reduced to – craving for these things that normal people don't even think about. The nurse brought the sheets in and tossed them on the bed. I changed the bed and went to my bag to put my clothes on the shelves. There were cigarette packets and butts on the shelves, and tobacco littered the shelves. So, I went back out. This was half an hour later and Cynthia and my mum had gone.

I said, 'You need to go in there and clean that room.'

They said, 'We're not cleaning it.'

I said, 'I'm not touching it, so you need to go in there and clean it.' Then **beep-beep-beep**. A nurse had hit the alarms because I was raising my voice. My senses screamed at me and the balloon in my head burst. They restrained me and gave me an injection. After the restraint, they left me on the floor. I got up when I was able to, went to the bed I had made and, heavy from sedation, fell into a deep sleep.

At midnight the lights went on. As brightness flooded my eyes, the black figures came towards me. It took a few seconds to realise I was being awoken for transfer back to PICU in a cage. Four hours earlier I had come in a taxi. Apparently, as my behaviour demonstrated, I hadn't been ready for transfer.

Cynthia wasn't here when I got back, but the following day she acknowledged what had happened, that was all. It took three more weeks to get out. Dr Saty discharged me home. That rarely happens. Usually people have to go back to acute. I think he realised acute wouldn't have been therapeutic. I didn't need another Clover experience.

I couldn't locate the distressing states I was having in anything I knew. I needed help. Professional help. And I wasn't getting it. Not in psychiatric units or the community. In the community I didn't cope. I kept getting readmitted as I engaged in sensory-seeking experiences such as walking at the side of motorways because I was attracted to lights and the sound of cars. Due to bed pressures (occupancy rates of beds are usually at 100%), I was merely contained in hospitals, the cause of my issues not investigated or addressed. With poor follow-up care I was doomed to be what the staff in the unit called a "revolving door" patient.

There were four moves in the next two months, all more of the same.

4–9 July 2013, Geranium Ward;

18 July–2 August 2013, PICU Ivy Suite. Discharged by Tribunal. Panel challenged diagnosis, stating it was Alexis's reaction to Josh's death.

10 August 2013, Columbine Ward;

30 August 2013, Kirby Ward, Queens Hospital.

Trigger Warning: This chapter contains references to self-harm.

CHAPTER 23

Judy

2nd September 2013

I had only been in Primrose a little while when I had an incident with an HCA named Judy. She was a talented, articulate, and clever woman. I used to get on with her very well. She was good at art, and often helped me with the technical aspects of my drawing. I had known her for nine months and so she would talk through with me what I had drawn. Just before the incident, she helped me draw a picture of Josh in his coffin. She was a good woman.

One day I said to Judy, 'I need to have some PRN medication.' PRN means "as needed". I could request extra meds when I felt I required them.

I felt like that balloon in my head was about to burst. So, I asked for the PRN. I needed the drug to stop overloads and meltdowns.

She said, 'Yes, Alexis. You can have the PRN medication after the staff handover to the oncoming shift at three o'clock.'

I told her, 'Okay, I'm going to wait for that.' The handover happened. The new staff came onto the ward. But the nurse was too busy to give me the meds. I said to Judy, 'It's three o'clock. What time can I expect to have the medication?' She told me I could have it in five minutes. So, it would be 3.05pm. I said, 'I can't have it at 3.05pm.' I didn't like fives. They're not a closed shape. I don't like odd numbers because of the sharp corners. Three isn't too bad because it's curvy, and you can stick the two bits together and get a circle. 'Can I have it at 3.06pm?'

'Yes, that's fine. It'll be about then.' Then it got to 3.06pm and she told me I couldn't have the medication because they weren't ready.

I was very frustrated. 'You need to let me have this medication because I need to go for a walk.'

Judy said, 'You can't have a walk because there's no nurse to take you for your Section 17 leave.' I could use my leave, because I had seven consecutive days of "good behaviour" and had used the leave properly every time, no running away.

I told her I'd been waiting the whole day. 'I just want my half-hour. I have 30 minutes a day. This is the time I always have it, every day at this time, so you need to let me out.'

She said, 'I can't let you out.'

So, I got very cross. The balloon in my head was getting too big. I couldn't understand why I couldn't have the PRN. And why couldn't I have my leave? It was very frustrating, and I didn't know why she was changing routines. I didn't know why the nurse was still in the office, because she was supposed to be doing the medication to let me go out. I didn't even want the medication, but I had to have it before I could go out.

I was by the exit door, and I told her, 'You need to let me out of the door.'

Judy said, 'Lexi, I'm not going to let you out the door.'

I said, 'Please, you need to let me out the door, please.' I was very polite to her. 'Because it's time. This is the time I have to go for my walk and I can't be late.'

She grabbed me just above my wrist.

I told her, 'Get off,' and pulled my arm away because the fire in my arm was agonising. She fell back against the wall.

She's fat, and she tripped over her foot. When she landed on the floor, she winded herself, had an asthma attack, and turned blue.

I was very stressed about that. I liked her a lot. The sight and sound of the incident was horrifying and haunts me. I ran into the ward to the sound of **beep-beep-beep**, into my room and wrapped myself up, covering my ears.

I caused her a lot of pain. Staff had to call an ambulance and she went to hospital. The staff told me these facts. They were so cross with me. I didn't get to go out. I called my mum. My mum phoned the ward and found out Judy had to have her leg in a cast. It was broken. She was alright. It was just a bad asthma attack.

I self-harmed. I didn't know how else to cope. My mum told the nurse, 'Alexis has cut herself.'

The nurse, Kimberley – who would help me design a tattoo on my arm to disguise all the scars the following year – told my mum she didn't want to speak to me, because she had feelings as well and she didn't want to attend to my cut. She was too cross with me in that moment.

So, my mum told her, 'You can either go help Alexis with that, or I'm going to come and do it myself.' So, Nurse Kimberley came, and she told me I was despicable.

Judy brought charges, but the police didn't follow up for three months. I was unaware the incident had even been reported. Judy had wanted to charge me with assault. I told the policeman, who came on New Year's Day to talk to me, that I didn't intentionally hurt Judy, that she had grabbed my arm and it hurt and I pulled away. My mum knew him, and he's known me since I was little.

When the policeman read me the story Judy told them, it was the same as my version of events. He said, 'It's not a crime. It's an incident that happened as a result of her intervention.' In the end the police report read, 'Not in the public interest to continue'.

CHAPTER 24

Auntie Ellen's Visit

My Auntie Ellen, an elderly lady, used to get the bus nine miles from Morecombe Cove to see me at Primrose. I had known her since I was a tiny baby and she used to babysit me sometimes when I was small. Auntie Ellen was a strong Christian women and I found her to be very accepting and non-judgemental. I used to enjoy her visits as, like many of the other occupants of psych wards, I didn't have many visitors. She always brought me a packet of Cadbury Freddo bars. I loved chocolate, so I was pretty excited to see her.

She was there when Leroy, the deputy ward manager, told me I would be moved to a PICU in London. The news was shocking and unexpected. When he informed me of the transfer, I cried in Auntie Ellen's lap for about an hour. She didn't talk and I didn't say anything. I was overwhelmed and my skin was prickling. She cuddled me and the pressure of her body felt good.

As she was leaving I told Leroy, 'I'm going to say goodbye to her.'

He said, 'You can't say goodbye to her.'

I told him, 'I always say goodbye to her. It's very rude if you don't say goodbye.' Knowing I wouldn't see her again for a long time as PICU was far away, I really insisted. It was unbearable being sent so many miles from home. It made me even more isolated and alone.

She went out through the airlock, and I tried to go with her but they grabbed me. In front of her, they smashed me onto the floor. She was screaming through the door window for them to get off. They pulled me into the calming room, which wasn't very calming. I was crying in there. Auntie Ellen lay next to me on the floor while I recovered from that. I didn't see her again. She was too traumatised to come to the ward. I don't blame her. And so that was one less visitor. One less human connection.

CHAPTER 25

My Mate Blair

Before my madness set in I had a made a new friend, Blair. This was quite an achievement for me and, needless to say, I didn't initiate the relationship. Blair was pushing her buggy on our road when my mum stopped her. I had tiny Abi in my arms and couldn't believe that Mum wanted to chat with another ex-criminal she knew from her police service. She was always doing that. We could hardly walk down the road without someone saying hello. This meant that I'd have to communicate and engage in social niceties.

In Blair's buggy was her baby daughter Susan. After some discussion, in which I initially feigned an interest, it turned out Blair was Mum's police colleague. And her mother had also served with my mother. Blair and I are the same age and our daughters were born a few days apart. According to my mother, with such "wonderful" commonalities, we obviously had to be friends. She invited Blair over to our house and within a few visits I could converse quite easily with her. We became friends. Usually on weekends because we were both working, together we would take our girls out.

Even during my madness, Blair was there. Like Auntie Ellen and a handful of other persons in my life, she didn't judge me. In fact, Blair didn't believe there was anything wrong with me. She agreed that I was different, but not ill. This made a significant difference to me in my darkest hours as I still had relationships in the world outside of psychiatry. It was refreshing to not only get out of the wards but also my parents' grasp. Because my mum trusted Blair, she didn't bother me too much when I wanted to go out with her. I knew Mum was worried about me, but I also needed some relief from her concern.

Blair and I would go to all sorts of places, usually outdoors. My favourite was a Country Park which hosted a cycling track. When I knew Blair and I were going to cycle with kids I looked up a few facts. I told her that in 2014, 18,844 cyclists were injured in reported road accidents, including 3,339 who were killed or seriously injured. She said she was pleased that we were going to a designated cycle path.

I thought, *Actually, mate, those figures only include cyclists killed or injured in road accidents that were reported to the police.* In fact, many cycling casualties are not reported. Although the number of deaths is accurate, there could be two or three times as many seriously injured cyclists and double the number of slightly injured. But I didn't say this. I just smiled at Blair.

Just as we were about to set off, Blair fell over in the car park. Susan was on the back of the bike. It was quite funny because it happened slowly like in a cartoon. Susan, from her perch on Blair's bike, looked at her mother mockingly. Blair's arm kept hurting though. She found out later that it was broken.

I guessed she wouldn't be reporting that injury to the police. I informed her that was why the figures I quoted were misleading. Blair said, 'That's good to know, Lexi.'

On a good day I am often subject to constant scrutiny because I am so different. I find myself constantly calibrating myself to fit in. It's exhausting.

Blair accepted me and my quirks.

CHAPTER 26

PICU Slade at Beckton

After Judy broke her foot, they sent me to a private PICU in London. I entered this ward feeling like the worst kind of human. I knew why I was there. The staff knew why I was there. Judy was a good woman. I had replayed in my head the image of what happened to her many times, watching her each time struggling for breath, screaming because of her ankle.

Ivy Suite didn't blame me. They acknowledged my story and the struggle I had. But I was punished. I challenged the assertion I was aggressive, that I had deliberately hurt poor Judy. The response I got from the Assistant Director of Acute Clinical Services confirmed I didn't mean to hurt her, or anybody else ever.

She wrote back to us on 17th November 2013:

Alexis has never attacked anyone … however she displays behaviour that puts herself at risk and potentially other people.

Judy had no reason to grab me. She probably thought that it would be fine, that it's just Lexi. Grab her on the arm and pull her back. But my act of pulling away, or as they put it, 'Alexis bent forwards, and then threw her body back therefore throwing Judy off', was the crime I have paid for over and over.

The NHS knew about my sensory reactions. I told them. I just had no diagnosis to back it up. That's a huge problem.

If you say, 'That hurts,' they'll say something like, 'Oh, yeah, well, you should think about your behaviour, then it wouldn't be an issue.' They don't listen, especially the doctors. The HCAs are more aware and compassionate because they have more time on the floor.

There were no beds in Ivy so they sought a private bed to transfer me quickly. Because the hospital was private and they wouldn't be swapping two patients, the NHS had to take the bed immediately. This meant there was no midnight transfer.

I told them I wasn't going. They said, 'This is why we tell you in the middle of the night, Lexi. Do you want to see Abi before you go?' I said yes. I went to the family room and had two hours with Abi and Mum and Dad before I left. Then we all walked out of Primrose together. There, right in front, was the ambulance, doors open, and a cage inside wide open. My mum, holding Abi, burst into tears, and broke down.

My dad was saying, 'Come on, Beth. Come on, Beth. Let's get to the car.'

She said, 'I can't.' She just froze, looking at the cage.

Staff told me, 'Just get in the ambulance.' So, I jumped in, and off we went.

It was Deputy Ward Manager Craig, of the "Fucking Bitch Disorder" comment, doing the transfer. We had a nice chat all the way there. That was the furthest I had travelled in a cage. It was a good three hours before we arrived in London.

The hospital was on a deprived council estate inside a tall perimeter fence. I'd never been in such a place. My only reaction was, 'Oh.'

Craig said, 'Oh, gosh.'

I asked him, 'Have you been here before, Craig?' He said no.

Before I entered I looked up the PICU on the Care Quality Commission website. The CQC is an organisation which regulates and inspects hospitals. This PICU was rated as "Inadequate". Great!

The cage was opened while Craig met with two uniformed nurses from the PICU. Craig didn't shake their hands. As we went inside, I realised I was walking into bedlam. There was no other way to describe it.

In Ivy Suite there was discipline because the staff were in charge. Here, the women seemed to run the place. Staff had barricaded themselves in the familiar glass office. The patients were at the glass, banging and banging. Craig just looked at me. I said, 'Don't leave me here, Craig,' and burst into tears. I'd never seen anything like it.

There was a lady there named Jean, whom I recognised from Primrose. She yelled, 'Hi, Lex! How are you doing?' Every other word that came out of her mouth was "fuck" or "cunt". She was a very tough woman, about 60, with long, unkempt blonde hair. Her teeth were black and rotted. But she was a lovely person. She took care of me in there.

Jean told me, 'I've been in here a few days, Lexi. You need to be tough or they're going to beat you up.'

I said, 'I think I'll be alright, Jean. I'm 6'1".'

She said, 'No, really, Lex. It's dangerous in here. This is London, innit? It's London.' I smiled, thinking she was exaggerating.

Staff put me straight on a 1:1 obs. On the first night before bed, the HCA who was on the obs said, 'You need to stay in your room. You'll get attacked.'

When I was taken off the 1:1 after 48 hours, a tiny blonde girl walked up to me and slapped me on the face.

Jean saw her, rushed over and grabbed her by the hair, threw her on the floor, and kicked her. Jean yelled, 'Don't you touch my friend, you fucking cunt.' There was no staff to help. But this little woman never touched me again.

When I wanted to call home, which was often, the staff had to open the door to their precious office and pass out a phone on a cord, then shut the door. I would sit on the floor outside the office as distressed women hammered on the window above me demanding things.

You were only supposed to have one call a day. People waited in line, shouting, 'Get off the fucking phone.' I would only talk to my dad when I was on this ward because my mum couldn't bear it. Crying, I begged him, 'Dad, you've got to get me out of here.' He could hear the screaming, yelling, and fighting through the phone. He phoned Gabriel, the service manager for the hospital, every day at nine o'clock in the morning and five o'clock in the evening insisting I have better treatment and that I was transferred.

I wasn't sleeping at all. It seemed the patients were sedated so that half were awake in the day and the other half at night. This made sense as staff had to deal with only half the ward at a time. I was constantly crying, and even prayed to God. I don't believe in God but I thought I would try everything.

One day, an HCA came to my door. 'Yes?' I said, peeking through the window slats.

She said, 'Alexis, I'm going off shift now.'

I said, 'Okay.' I didn't care who was on shift.

The HCA said, 'I'm not supposed to tell you, but there's a woman who's just been admitted from a prison nearby. She's very violent, and she hates white people.' Jean and I were the minority ethnic group on the ward. Jean would be fine. Even though I have a black belt in martial arts, I couldn't hurt a fly. It's just not in me.

The HCA said, 'I'm going to lock the door, and I'm going to pray for you. I hope you're okay in the morning.'

I checked the now-locked door, closed the slats, and cried. I couldn't believe how I had gotten here. It was another all-time low.

After a traumatic few days, I saw the RC, named Dr Adio. He was a petite African man who always wore a bow tie. He was gentle, softly spoken, and had a lovely manner about him.

He spent some time with me, and after his assessment he said, 'You don't have a personality disorder. You have Adjustment Disorder, AD.'

I looked it up. I seemed to relate to this diagnosis much more than EUPD. Adjustment Disorder is caused by a stressor. I had no specific problems before, which led me to agree. AD linked directly to my bereavement with Josh. Dr Adio told me I should have recovered from Josh's death within six months, which is normal for most people. I had failed to adjust in the correct way and hadn't followed the usual grieving process. I agreed that I was impaired in social, occupational, and all the other areas of functioning, so I thought his diagnosis was correct.

I think now how close he was to the truth. My failure to respond "normally" to grief is part of autism. He was so close, and he'd only known me for seven days.

In the final meeting I had with Dr Adio, he said, 'Your dad has applied, through your solicitor, for next-of-kin discharge.' In England, once every six months the next of kin has the legal right to order discharge unless the threshold is too high, or unless I'm an immediate danger to myself or others, which I clearly wasn't. Dr Adio discharged me. It was a great day!

I left the hospital with my discharge paperwork and a new diagnosis of AD. My dad's persistent telephoning to Gabriel worked. I am not sure I would've gotten out so quickly without him.

CHAPTER 27

Freezing in Seclusion

28th October 2013

I was in the community for six weeks after I was discharged from Slade PICU. I wasn't coping well with the trauma from my time in the Beckton. I would wake up in such terror having flashbacks. I thought I was still in the unit. It would take a good hour to calm down and re-orientate myself to being home. I was overwhelmed by everything that had happened. I took a drug overdose and was admitted to Quince Ward.

On 30th October in the ward round, I met my new RC, Dr Williams. He suggested they extend my Section 2, under which I was being assessed for 28 days, turning it into a Section 3, so they could keep me for six more months of treatment. He also asked why I hadn't succeeded at suicide yet! Why didn't I just take more drugs when I overdosed? Actually, the most effective concoction I knew well, having researched it. I didn't want to die. I just didn't know how to manage the overload. I didn't know what was going on with me, why my brother had died or how I had gotten into this terrible state. Overdosing gave me a break from the relentless helplessness and distress I felt. At least in the short term.

Dr Williams's comments created a cognitive overload for me. I tried to calm myself as I struggled to manage the explosion in my brain. In an impulsive and panicked way, I headed to the toilet, my skin prickling. I took a bin bag and wrapped it around me. I felt my skin relax as the pressure from the swaddle gave me feedback. I covered my eyes too, so the lights were not so bright. I breathed easy, feeling secure.

When staff came in to find me, they immediately activated the alarm. They picked me up, and that hurt a lot. I tried to get them off me. I used my body to wriggle free. Their tight grips were the hurt you get when you're being bruised. They carried me like a battering ram to the seclusion room. It took nine of them, as I writhed like a snake to get away.

In seclusion, they crashed me down onto the blue mattress, pressing me into it. I had trouble breathing. They pulled my trousers off and removed my jumper. They held first one side of my face onto the mat, then the other, as they removed my earrings. Two injections in the butt, and they left. I hadn't been in this room before – three white walls and one window.

It was very cold. Two HCAs were looking at me through the window slits. We made eye contact and they closed the blinds. Nice, I thought. It wasn't long before my heart rate settled and I realised it was very, very cold.

I begged them, 'Please, I'm so cold.' The air conditioning was coming in full blast. I liked its steady hum of noise, though. Soon I needed to sleep, but the bare plastic mattress was too cold to lie on.

I knocked on the window, crying to them, 'Please, I'm too cold.' They had taken my clothes off. I just had my bra, underpants, and a vest top, but no trousers. I was freezing.

It wasn't long before even my feet were so cold it hurt to stand up. I was shivering. I tucked my hands in my armpits, periodically rubbing them together.

I showed the HCAs my nails through the window, 'Look, they're turning blue. Give me a blanket, please. Or just turn the air con down.'

When I knocked on the window, sometimes they ignored me. Sometimes they peeked through the blinds. Eventually they showed me the thermometer through the window. It read 21 degrees. I said, 'That's 21 in your room, not in this room.' They're not supposed to talk to you, and they didn't. I got a shrug, which I interpreted as, 'Whatever'.

Here's their version, dated 30th October 2013:

Staff were finding it very difficult to establish any holds because Alexis was very sweaty after struggling with staff for so long, eventually due to her being totally uncooperative, it took nine staff to move her up the corridor and then myself, RJ, MS, TS, YZ, TR, FD, placed her onto the seclusion room mattress and then staff retreated using PSTS technique. Alexis then charged towards the door but staff managed to close it in time. While in seclusion, Alexis has periodically asked myself and HCA JJ to open the door and to give her a blanket and then some clothes because she was feeling "cold". The temperature has been a constant 21 Degrees Centigrade according to the seclusion room thermometer ...

I was in turmoil because I had never encountered the problem of a freezing room. I knew that I needed to sit still because if I moved too much, I'd look agitated. However, if I was still, I was too cold.

It was a conundrum. I recalled the time I was bored in seclusion and did a full circuit workout. That was a long seclusion due to my "agitation". This was different though. I decided to alternate between sitting and standing. I tried to do each for about 30 minutes. I thought that would satisfy them, and also my need to keep some areas of my body warm.

I remembered the survival training from my outdoor education class. So, I sat on my bum and crossed my legs. I put my knees under my vest top, and wrapped my arms around me. I was shivering badly. I worked it out by counting all the minutes to be about half an hour. I would count to 60 because I like the number six. Then I would get up and knock, and politely ask for something, and they would always say no.

When staff were satisfied by my presentation, a nurse entered the room to assess me. She said, 'Goodness, Alexis. It's freezing in here.'

My whole body was shivering when I came out. I said, 'I know it's freezing. I've been telling those HCAs for hours.' But I was too cold to argue. The nurse put blankets around me – the kind made of foil. They gave me very hot tea in a porcelain mug, which I hadn't had for a long time. My fingernails and my lips were pale. Staff stayed with me and monitored my temperature. It took a long time to go back to normal. I had been in there for six hours, and I was still freezing after 45 minutes.

They didn't take me back to the ward but had the doctor check me. I was held in the communal part of the seclusion suite, and the service manager, Ms Davies, came in all apologetic. I was really annoyed, but also sedated and still recovering.

I later wrote a letter to the CEO, to complain. She wrote back on 12th November 2013:

You may recall that Ms Davies met with you to apologise on the day and again we offer our sincere apologies for your experience and the coldness of the room. This should not have happened and as a service, we are deeply saddened and appalled that this did. The staff who were monitoring you in the seclusion room were recording the temperature, and clearly the system was not working and was giving a false reading. Ms Davies immediately asked that our estates and facilities colleagues look into this and rectify the situation. The 136 suite, in which the seclusion room is located, has been approved for a full upgrade and this will include a redesign of the seclusion room which will consist of a whole new temperature control system that maintains a constant, comfortable temperature. Please be assured that this does not mean that we are not addressing the system in the meantime.

The CEO missed the point. If they were really saddened and appalled, they would have disciplined the two staff whom I begged and begged, the two staff who watched me shiver for six hours. They should have called the estate manager when I was trying in vain to get warm, not wait until I was out! I'm not the least bit interested in the full upgrade and refurbishment of their unit. I have flashbacks about my time in that room. The damage to my psyche is enduring.

They wrote:

Severity and Result

Did this incident result in harm? No harm caused as a result of this incident.

Seriously! No harm was caused! – Well ... thanks for saying sorry ...

CHAPTER 28

Sexual Assault

24th December 2013

This ward, Radcliffe, was part of the same hospital as Ivy Suite PICU. The day I was transferred, my mum arrived with my brother Thomas to visit me. They asked me, 'Lexi, have you been out of your room?' I told them I hadn't. I'd been there six or seven hours, and it was after lunch. It had been too noisy for me to leave.

My mum said, 'Do you know where to get your dinner, Lexi?' I told her I didn't.

She said to the nurse, 'Why hasn't she left her room? She doesn't even know where to go to get food. Why haven't you shown her around?'

The nurse said, 'Oh, we were just too busy.' So, the nurse went with my mum, my brother, and me. While I was looking around, my mum noticed this guy was following us. I would later learn that his name was Ian.

Visiting time was only an hour. It was tough because the ward was far from our family home and it took my mum an hour and a half to drive there. After they left I was sitting in my room, and Ian came inside and sat on the desk. I had put my clothes at the back of the desk shelf so I had space to draw.

I kept my drawing implements immaculate. The pencils were always sharpened well in case I needed to draw. And I made sure they were the same length all the way along, even though the black had to be a lot shorter. I had nice pencils.

Ian was sitting there, just looking at me and occasionally talking. I didn't think that was strange because I didn't understand about behaviour like that. Even now I don't really. It was dinnertime, and he asked me, 'Do you want to go and have some food?' I told him I didn't want to have any food.

He said, 'Just come with me.' He took me along what I had remembered to be the long corridor out of the units. It was the door that joined all the wards together. It was also a dead end.

I told him, 'Ian, I've been here before. This corridor leads to another unit.'

He said, 'No, it doesn't.' I had a poor cognitive map and wasn't processing at all well so I trusted him.

He went to the door and it was locked. He pushed me face forward against the door. Pressing me into the door, he pulled up my top and was trying to pull down my trousers. His whole body was pressing on mine. For a moment, I was frozen. I couldn't move or shout out. Feeling his hot body on mine and his breathing on my neck paralysed me. I felt him rubbing his penis on my back.

It felt like forever, but it couldn't have been that long until I became oriented. I thought I would probably get free. But I didn't know what to do. The pressure of his body, the loud breathing and the slimy, wet, and sticky feeling was all I could think of, overwhelming me. Then when I realised what was happening, I twisted away and ran. I shouted and screamed.

I ran into the female ward and found Chloe, a nurse. I told her what had happened. She kept trying to cut me off, telling me I was on the wrong ward and needed to go to back to Radcliffe. She called Radcliffe and a male nurse came over. I told them everything. I said I couldn't go back. Nurse Chloe showed me off the ward. I felt dirty. I was hot and sweaty. Now I had to go back there, to that ward, where he was.

I told the Radcliffe nurse I was upset. I was just about to say it was because of Ian when he cut me off and said I shouldn't come back inside the ward until I had calmed down and felt safe. How silly. Of course I didn't feel safe. That wouldn't improve in the next 15 minutes or 15 hours.

I entered the ward, running to my room in case I saw Ian. I tied a knot in the end of a blanket, threw the knot over the top of my door and shut the door. This kept the blanket from sliding off the door. Then I wrapped the blanket round my neck and head. The noose provided much-needed pressure. I tried to calm. I started to orient myself and process.

Somebody pressed the alarm, **doot-doot-doot-doot**. They grabbed me, smashed me on the floor, jabbed me, and put me in the seclusion room for hours. Inside the room I was trying to come to terms with what had happened. If I was just better at understanding people, I might have avoided that guy. I was still sweaty and wet. I thought what I had done that made this happen was try to be a decent human by talking to Ian. I didn't know what he would do. I felt something so intensely inside like an embarrassment.

Why didn't staff listen? I was even trying to explain to them when they came in my room and on the way to seclusion.

I didn't feel safe at all. Not from the patients or the staff. This was supposed to be a place of recovery. I had told staff I didn't want Ian in my room, and they made out like I was being antisocial. So, I had talked to him.

Seclusion is a quiet and lonely place. All you have are your thoughts and yourself. I felt disgusting. What sort of vile human was I? I wanted to leave this room, leave this ward, and go somewhere I would be okay. But where was that? I didn't fit into this world. I was a strange anomaly. I couldn't even protect myself. I was not safe. I sat for hours with this going through my head, frightened.

I didn't know, but my mum was phoning up. They kept telling her, 'Alexis is busy at the moment. You can't speak to her right now.' She tried all day to reach me, and most of the next day.

I phoned her the next evening. She asked, 'Why didn't you phone me yesterday, Lexi? I've been trying to reach you for two days.'

I told her what happened. She said, 'Right. That's it.' She phoned Staff Nurse Rozi. She said, 'How dare you? How dare you? Why didn't you tell me about this?'

He said, 'There was no sexual assault. Nothing happened.' He was right, nothing about what had happened had been recorded in my notes.

She said, 'Alexis reported it to the nurse on the women's ward, and also to the male nurse on your ward.'

Nurse Rozi said, laughing, 'There is no record of that.' He was right, there was no record.

She said, 'How dare you laugh at me? What is funny about my daughter being sexually assaulted on your unit?'

He said, 'I'll get back to you when I have more information.'

Nurse Rozi called my mum later. 'There was no sexual assault because it wasn't reported.' My mum told him the names of the nurses. Because she had said their names, they had to acknowledge what she was saying. Chloe denied the interaction with me, as did the male nurse. I was told not to make "allegations".

I was upset and wished I had told no one. My mum called the police and I was interviewed. My mum insisted I was moved off this ward with 17 men. In my transfer notes, my new risk was that of "making allegations". My mum was stronger than me and told the staff, 'If you're not going to do something about it, then I am. I want my daughter moved off that ward in the next few hours because it's dangerous for her there.'

The police interviewed Ian. He admitted much of what he had done. He said he "fancied" me. The police were not able to prosecute or do much as he was deemed not to have sufficient capacity. So, nothing happened to him. And worst of all nothing happened to the staff who lied. Who do people believe? Not a crazy mental patient like me.

CHAPTER 29

Felicity Hart

4th February 2014

I finally got back to Blackthorn hospital in Heysham and was put in Primrose. I had just left PICU again. I wasn't improving. The doctors were hesitant to take what they thought was a risk by removing the section. The treatment I received made me worse, but I also didn't do well during discharge because I was in utter turmoil. The crazy thing is you must be in hospital a long time before you get psychology and / or specialist placement.

Dr Felicity Hart, the wonderful clinical psychologist was doing her best to help me. Felicity looked like she just stepped out of a time machine from the '60s. She wore spectacles that made her eyes look bigger than they were. Her hair was long and was always plaited, and she wore baggy hippy clothes. Felicity had a son with autism. She was also trained in DBT (Dialectical Behaviour Therapy) so she was very empathetic and caring. She wasn't put off by my diagnosis of EUPD and didn't treat me badly because of it. She was also sensitive to my need to know what would happen and how it might happen. Felicity had a way of reducing my anxiety.

I saw her once a week. She taught me the basics of DBT, never to look at the past, but focus on how I could manage here and now. She prepared me for many changes on the ward. I am most indebted to her for how she assisted me with the forensic assessment. Apparently, I was now forensic material and I was petrified. Such services are reserved for those who exhibit extremely challenging and dangerous behaviours who have usually had contact with the criminal justice system. I talked to Dr Hart about it.

She said, 'Alexis, these are many things you could say and do to achieve the goal you want.' I interpreted this statement to mean, 'This is how you can get out of the situation.'

I didn't think forensic services would help and I like to believe that Dr Hart didn't either. We made notes and she helped prepare me mentally for what felt like a life-changing exam with the forensic doctor. We practised what I would say to the doctor. His name was Dr Omar Hussein, from London.

I asked staff, 'Please, can you tell me when the forensic doctor is coming, please?' Anyway, they didn't tell me. So, at three o'clock one day, this man turns up. They called me. It was too noisy so I was in my room.

They said, 'This is Dr Omar Hussein.' He was a small, skinny man. He looked like he was from the Emirates, a Muslim guy. He came and shook my hand and held it for a long time. This was another example of unnecessary physical contact. We did the forensic assessment. He told me he did not think I was suitable for a forensic service. Thank fuck!

But Dr Dempsey, the RC who initially was responsible for my care when I first became dysregulated, wasn't satisfied or happy with that. She needed Dr Hussein's approval to get rid of me. He had said no. Dr Dempsey contacted my community nurse and told her to 'Update the referral form, risk assessment and care plan ... requesting that Dr Omar Hussein send to St Andrews an updated report that recommends a low / medium secure unit'. So, St Andrews, a huge bed provider for forensic services in the South of England, sent their man. I said the same stuff to him.

He said I was very suitable and there was a bed for me on their locked personality disorder unit.

I was petrified! 'Felicity, they're trying to send me to medium secure hundreds of miles from home, with a 5.2-metre perimeter fence, and no leave. I'll never see my daughter.'

She said, 'Have a look at other options, Alexis.' I found a great personality disorder hospital in York called The Retreat.

Dr Hart said, 'Perfect, you'll have autonomy, be able to have your say, create your own care pathways. That sounds better. DBT-focused – excellent. Good find, Alexis. Now convince them.'

I contacted The Retreat to get their policies for referral and sent them a letter. Dr Hart helped, as did my community psychiatric nurse.

Soon after, I was called for an interview. They were kind, polite, and quick to respond. This is unusual. It's normally the case that as the recipient of "care", you don't matter. This place was different.

Dr Dempsey wouldn't let me go. She cancelled my first appointment, saying I was too much of a risk. Then my mum got involved.

She called Dr Dempsey and told her she would drive me to York herself. Mum said, 'Look, they called her for an assessment. We'll drive her if you don't have the staff. We'll be responsible. You just write up her leave.' They didn't want to be responsible if I absconded. In the end, Dr Dempsey didn't have a choice. She had to try the least restrictive option. I don't think she believed I would be accepted.

CHAPTER 30

Assessment for York

I went up to York. It was a huge stately home with acres of manicured gardens. It was just incredible. All the doors were open. There were no locks. I walked in and breathed a huge sigh of relief. The corridors were very narrow, like rabbit runs, turn this way, go this way, through this door. The floorboards were all creaky. Everything about the place felt wonderful.

My mum was equally impressed. We were treated with respect and dignity. It wasn't something she was used to, either. Sitting in the waiting room next to a huge grandfather clock, my mum was smiling, and urged me to do well in the interview so I could come to this place.

The doctor was on time. Little things like this meant so much. I was worth keeping time for. He shook my hand and said, 'My name is Charlie.' His manner was warm.

I said, 'It's nice to meet you, doctor.'

He smiled reassuringly and said, 'No, no. Here in The Retreat we use a flattened hierarchy. Your word is just as important as mine, so call me Charlie.' Being spoken to that way, after more than a year of being treated like shit, was refreshing.

He showed me to his office. There were no other staff there. He didn't think I was a ticking time bomb, nor did anyone check to be sure Charlie was still alive. For one long hour, we were uninterrupted. He asked questions and then listened to my answers. I acknowledged my struggles and predicament. He reassured me there was hope. After the interview, I had lunch with The Retreat community.

In a therapeutic community, everyone works together to achieve goal-orientated recovery. Each group member's voice is important – this is a participative group-based approach. Part of the interview was the community interviewing you.

I visited the rooms where the clients slept, as well as the kitchen and therapy rooms. Outside each room was a printed sheet that read:

Turn up, Tune in, Tell the Truth.

Now I wanted more than ever to go to this hospital. I didn't think I would ever say I wanted to be in hospital, but this place was different.

The community interview was tough. The clients grilled me. The programme is for women with self-defeating behaviours, so their questions were, 'Do you light fires? Do you ligature?' It was hard to be asked these questions so openly by peers. I didn't know what to say. I wasn't prepared for the intensity. I remembered the sign outside. I had turned up, I was tuned in and I told the truth. The clients were non-judgemental. I had never experienced such ... acceptance?

There was a nurse in the room but she might as well not have been there. The interview was run by the clients.

After the interview, I had a chat with one of the staff. They said they would be in touch with my community psychiatric nurse. I had a walk around the gardens, and eagerly told my mum everything. I thought I had done well, and was hoping for a place there.

After four or five hours, we drove home. I'd had the whole day off the ward and it had gone well. Then I walked back in through the Primrose airlock. Bang! Through the next airlock. Bang! I thought, what is this all about? Is this effective?

Then it all kicked off. As soon as I walked in, I was greeted not by a calm tranquillity, but by noise and chaos. I panicked inside. I knew even if I was accepted, I couldn't go to York because I was on a section. I had to negotiate the sensory assault every day and get the section removed. This would be tough.

Thankfully, I had a tribunal coming up. A tribunal is a legal hearing that takes place in an informal setting at hospital. This tribunal had the power to discharge me from section, recommend that I get to leave and transfer me to another hospital. Tribunals happen once every six months. It was super-lucky that mine was coming up because St Andrews, the medium secure unit, had already accepted me.

If I got the section removed, I would avoid St Andrews. By law, The Trust must take the least restrictive option. The stakes were high. As Nurse Achala from Ivy PICU always said, 'It's all in your hands, Lexi.' I felt pressure. I was determined to manage this better. I needed to talk to Dr Hart. I had a goal and hope, more than I'd had in a long time.

CHAPTER 31

Assessment for York

My solicitor Jessica Abbott and I prepared hard for the tribunal. The tribunal panel is a judge, a doctor, and a layperson. Before the hearing, Jessica and the panel members get three reports: a medical report from Dr Dempsey, a nursing report from my named nurse on Primrose Eva, and a social circumstances report from my community psychiatric nurse. The reports help them determine whether I should be discharged from the hold of the Mental Health Act.

We went through the nursing report and Jessica prepared questions to ask the nurse in the cross-examination. We went through the social circumstances report. I wasn't too concerned about this one, as my parents were at the tribunal and would help answer questions in a positive way. The important piece, however, was the doctor's report. We hadn't received it so we couldn't prepare our defence. I was worried.

The day before the tribunal, Jessica contacted me. She still had no report from the doctor. She questioned whether Dr Dempsey was coming. Dr Dempsey caused me concern because I knew she didn't want my section removed. She would fight hard to keep it in place. She could have removed the section and sent me to York. But no report, no doctor – what was going on?

The day of the tribunal I walked off the unit to the designated room. We waited outside in the lovely spring air. Eva was also there, because I'm so dangerous, and Jessica as well as my CPN (Community Psychiatric Nurse). Inside the tribunal room sat the judge at the middle of a long table. On his left was the medical officer who was a psychiatrist, and on his right somebody with knowledge of medicine or psychiatry like a social worker. We were all there, but the bloody doctor hadn't shown up.

The judge and his people were on the opposite side of the table from us. We were supposed to walk in and seat ourselves – first the doctor, then the solicitor, then me, then the social worker. But since there was no doctor, we couldn't go in. We waited outside.

Eventually, Dr Pumba, a more inexperienced psychiatrist who worked closely with Dr Dempsey, showed up. He was always smiling. He hadn't even been able to write my prescription properly. I had to have it rewritten three times because he couldn't spell the medication. I was actually pleased to see him because he was nowhere near as strong and able as Dr Dempsey. I felt better about this situation already.

Dr Pumba knocked on the tribunal door after ignoring all of us outside, and said to the panel that because I hadn't allowed him to speak to me, he didn't write a report until this morning. This was a load of crap.

I was thinking, *This is a legal hearing where they will determine whether I'm locked up for five years, and you lie, then don't even write a report until the morning of the tribunal? He should have submitted his report much earlier so Jessica and I could prepare our defence. He didn't even bring it. He told the panel that he would go and print it because he'd just finished writing. Right,* I thought. *You didn't write it in time. You don't care about my future and you are playing games.* The panel was frustrated with him. He looked disorganised and unprofessional. Dr Pumba wandered off smiling to print the report.

Jessica told them, 'This is really unfair. We don't want to adjourn because of the stakes with Alexis's placement for York. Would you please give us an hour to look through the report?'

Dr Pumba came back with the report, and Jessica and I went out to look through it. It had the usual spelling errors and some manipulation of facts. Jessica got her questions ready, and I finally felt like we were prepared.

Then we all filed in. First, the panel questioned Dr Pumba. He told them how dangerous and aggressive I am. He cited Judy and the incident in Quince Ward as examples. I am an absconding risk, etc, etc.

The panel asked him about what he planned to do with me. What treatment was he planning for my awful conditions he had just described? He said I needed containment. They pressed him repeatedly. He was uncomfortable and stuttered and stammered. The medical doctor questioning him had spoken to me in the pre-tribunal interview. I gave him my version of events.

Dr Pumba finally caved under the pressure and finished his testimony by stating, 'We absolutely aren't sending Alexis to St Andrews.' He told them the placement would be inappropriate. I was stunned. And worried. *They might believe him,* I thought, then they won't discharge me. *What if they believe him and trust him?* At this point, Jessica was looking at him like, *you fucking liar.*

The panel continued to press him as he kept changing his perspective. They asked, 'Is she dangerous and needs a forensic placement, or can she go to a therapeutic community?'

Dr Pumba finally answered them coherently. 'No, no. We don't think it's right that she should go to a forensic facility. She really wouldn't be suitable for that. But we must have her on section because she's a real danger to herself. We need to control when she goes out. She wouldn't take her medication if she wasn't on section. So, we're not going to send her to St Andrews, but we need to have her on section.'

The panel psychiatrist and the judge looked at each other, and asked Dr Pumba again, 'But what's her treatment option, then? Forensic is a serious escalation if you think she can actually go to a therapeutic community – the two are quite different, Dr Pumba.'

Dr Pumba said, 'Oh, she can go to York.'

'But that's for informal patients and you have said she's dangerous.'

'Yes, yes. But we absolutely must have her on section. She is dangerous.'

Again the judge says, 'Yes, but she needs to be informal if she's going to York. And you can't send somebody dangerous to a community-based placement. So, let me understand this. You don't think she should go to St Andrews?'

Dr Pumba said, 'Absolutely not. We're absolutely not going to do that.'

'But why does it say in your report from Dr Dempsey that she's been accepted into a bed in St Andrews if you were not thinking of sending her there?'

Pumba said, 'Yes, she has been accepted into a bed. I got the letter this morning. Her acceptance letter to St Andrews has just arrived and is on my desk.'

The judge was getting cross at this stage. He said, 'So, do you not think it's important that we see this letter?'

Dr Pumba was like, 'Uh, uh, shall I send someone to get it?'

The judge said, 'No, you go get it and bring it down here now.'

So Pumba went off and got the letter. The letter said, 'On your own recommendation we are accepting Alexis into our medium secure unit.' Pumba's denial was a complete lie.

The judge asked, 'If you weren't thinking of sending her to St Andrews, why has she been accepted into a bed?'

When Jessica had her turn to cross-examine him, she got to the point. She was skilled in an inoffensive and quiet way.

No one could ever call her aggressive in her approach, but I know her to be an expert passive aggressive. Her direct questioning was not obvious. 'Dr Pumba, you don't think Alexis suitable for St Andrews. Is that right?'

'Yes,' he said.

'You are aware that she needs to be off section to go to York so you would have to remove her detention. Are you willing to do that? Are you willing to take Alexis off section to go to York?'

He said that he would not remove the section. Now it was clear to everyone that Dr Pumba did not understand.

The panel said, 'Right, okay. We're going to remove Alexis from section. We do not feel that she meets the criteria for detention, so she can go to York where she is happy to receive treatment.' They wished me well. And for the first time in a long time I felt truly hopeful.

CHAPTER 32

The Long Wait for a Bed

Then my life got a lot better. I had to wait six or seven weeks before York had a bed and could accept me. The tribunal put a condition on discharge that I remain in hospital informally until transfer. At least this gave me some freedom.

One of the best things was having more flexible leave. Because the hospital was on large grounds, and it was April, whenever I wanted I could sit on the grass with the squirrels, the trees, the birds, and the blossoms. Often, my mum brought a picnic and Abi, and we sat outside. I looked up at this beautiful tree with blossoms on it and said, 'If I had been in St Andrews, I would have missed that.' Abi sat on my lap, blissfully unaware of where she was and why. We were quite happy.

How can you go between such extremes, from being locked inside a 5.2-metre perimeter fence, or having a picnic whenever you like, all based on the lies of a doctor? If my solicitor wasn't so good, I don't know what would have happened. This played on my mind. But it wasn't helpful so I tried to focus on the present.

I didn't have many meltdowns before my transfer because I had a lot of freedom. If I was re-sectioned, I couldn't go to York. Felicity knew that so she used her whole team to help me. I had three or four hours of psychology sessions per week until I left.

Felicity had Luke and Reggine, two other Blackthorn hospital based therapists, give me more support and techniques to help manage. I was able to use them because I wasn't under section and had room to manoeuvre. I knew I was going somewhere good. My mind settled a lot knowing for the first time I would get therapy.

Luke, the young Greek therapist with jet black hair, helped me with emotions. He wore a capsule wardrobe which I loved. It was a black shirt, a skin-tight cardigan, and tight trousers, usually jeans. On his right finger, Luke had an infinity band tattoo. I asked him one day what it was. He said, 'It can mean whatever you want it to mean, Alexis.' Such a psychologist thing to say.

Luke did psychodynamic therapy. I thought it was a waste of time at first, to be honest. But after working with it, I started to understand a bit about emotions. It was the first time I had ever connected with my emotions. I didn't know any feelings I was experiencing. Luke changed that.

He might ask, 'What's happening to you? How do you feel?'

My answer would be, 'I'm sitting in this room on a chair.' For me, this sort of therapy is super-hard. I don't get it and it's frustrating. But he was very skilled. He stepped in a lot. By the end, every time I saw him, I would cry for 10 minutes. I don't understand what he did, but he did something. I've never been like that with anybody else.

The best bit of practical help was from Reggine. She had Asperger's. Reggine was tall and dressed in loose clothing like me. She wasn't one for love and happiness. She was different to Luke. Reggine was practical and hands-on. She was the first to spot my sensory sensitivities, so she put together what was called a sensory diet.

Reggine made an hourly timetable. At the start of every hour, I had to do 15 minutes of jumping on a trampoline, skipping, and doing lots of forward rolls down the corridor, as well as rocking and spinning and push-ups. I had done this before on my own, but I got in trouble for it. Now I was allowed to do it. It made a huge difference. Everything calmed down. None of us knew this before.

One day, I asked Reggine how she figured out about my sensory needs. She said that Felicity had shown her a picture I had drawn in art therapy. It was just me floating above the ground because everything was hurting. She asked about that when she first saw me. I told her, 'It's because everything is painful, Reggine. The sounds hurt. There's nothing in the picture that hurts my eyes.' Because she had Asperger's, she recognised it. Once again, I felt lucky.

I read the report two months later that Reggine wrote to York. In it, she said she thought I was on the autistic spectrum. She hadn't shared that information with me. But there was no point in doing anything about it at that stage because I was going to get some therapy.

For those six weeks, I was the most settled I had ever been, and would ever be, on an acute unit. This was the most settled I'd ever be in the system. Hope was re-instilled. I had leave to go home. I had the sensory diet. I realised that when somebody kicked off, I could do those exercises in my room. In the entire six weeks I spent there, I had few meltdowns or sensory overload. Amazing what some therapy could do!

If I'd had this at the start, would I have been okay? I tried not to think too much about that, because I'm sure the answer was yes.

CHAPTER 33

Two Tales of Student Nurse Georgia

Even though things were looking hopeful, I was still me. My brain hadn't changed and staff still saw my behaviour as volitional.

I remember one day well. It strikes me as remarkable how an event involving several people can be recalled and reported on so differently. I was informal and about to go for a walk. That the doors were always locked did not contradict the ward being considered open.

Overloaded that day, I desperately needed my walk. The staff, as usual, were very busy. I didn't want to disturb them, but I had to have someone let me out. There were three doors between me and the outside world. After a while I asked a couple of nurses. Have you ever heard of a "nurse's minute"? It's never 60 seconds. Their 'One minute, Alexis' was always 5 to 10 minutes at best.

A student nurse, Georgia, was on the ward. She said, 'Yes' to going out. We exited the first of three doors. We were now both in the airlock heading out into the sunny, cold day. For an hour, I had set my mind on this walk, and had planned my route, one of six routes I usually took. This involved six rounds of an area of the picturesque hospital grounds. In my mind my next 18–20 minutes were fixed. I knew what I was doing and had a sense of calm.

Just as we approached the second door of the 15-metre-long airlock, Georgia turned to me, holding the key card to get out. She looked at me and smiled as she told me she couldn't let me out. My insides crushed. My heart was beating hard, as though it needed to escape my chest. I managed to sputter, 'What?'

'You are not allowed out,' Georgia said. I was totally confused. Firstly, I should have been allowed out. I was an unrestricted patient. Secondly, she told me I could go out, so what had happened in the last 30 seconds to change her mind? Thirdly, why on earth was she smiling at me? And finally, why was she holding her key card up in the air? These things were overwhelming. My brain was so full up I thought it might explode before I could figure this out. The walls of the airlock seemed to glare at me. The strip lights on the ceiling were like full-beam headlights. I panicked.

Georgia laughed as she walked by me back to the first door. All I could think about was getting out to do my six rounds. Each round would take three minutes and 3 x 6 = 18. I would have been back before 20 minutes had passed. I had planned the walk and I needed to do it. Georgia was laughing at me.

I was so full. I managed, 'Let me out.' She said no, and kept laughing.

'What the fuck are you laughing at?' These words came out of my mouth before I even realised what I was saying. She ran off up the ward. I ran after her. I had to get out.

Walk of six

Six rounds

Each round will take three minutes

3 x 6 = 18.

Walk of six

Six rounds

Each round will take three minutes

3 x 6 = 18.

I followed her. I was panicking. My plan was falling apart. I was trapped. I couldn't get out. My plan was falling apart. My plan was falling apart.

Georgia didn't answer me and slammed the office door in my face. I kicked it. I didn't realise I had kicked it until my foot made contact with the door. My body, for this split second, felt okay. But as the feeling passed, my sense of awareness passed too. I was lost in space and time and I was terrified. I needed the feedback pressure of a hard surface so I could again locate myself.

Then the alarms sounded. My ears were hurting so badly. I screamed. I jumped to calm myself. Staff came running at me. I didn't have time to realise they were coming for me. At that moment, I felt on fire. My head had exploded, I couldn't think, I couldn't see, and my skin burnt. I was in agony. I tried to break free to run, to move and breathe. I could do none of these things.

Sometime later, I started to see faces. I felt hands on my skin. I was soaking wet. My chest and face pressed against floor. I felt the pressure of bodies on mine. My trousers and my underpants were dishevelled on my body. I could feel pain in my bottom. I panicked again as I looked into the eyes of the nurse holding my arm. I quickly averted my gaze. I heard voices. One was the voice of the nurse pressing my head. I didn't know what she was saying.

Time passed. I knew I had been injected. My voice was hoarse. I must have been shouting or screaming. I could feel the drugs in my body. I realised my wrist was throbbing. I remembered what had happened. As the staff got off me, I tried to explain that I needed to walk.

Walk of six

Six rounds

Each round will take three minutes

3 x 6 = 18.

I tried to explain to them about Georgia. They didn't want to hear it. They were angry.

Walk of six

Six rounds

Each round will take three minutes

3 x 6 = 18.

I kept thinking this. It calmed me.

I stopped. I don't know if it was me or the drugs, but I stopped. I started to cry. I hugged myself. I felt naked and scared.

I spent some time in the calming room. I didn't get a chance to explain. I tried to speak to nurses and HCAs but they didn't want to talk. That was fine. A day later, I think I was able to speak to a caring doctor.

*

Later, my named nurse, Eva, explained to me Georgia's side of the story, so different from mine. I told her Georgia was lying. I apologised to Georgia through staff for the "effect" I'd had on her. I didn't want anyone to be upset or scared. After I finally could explain, this was written in my risk status:

Risk: Agitation and aggression. Self-harming behaviour. Allegatory [sic] *behaviour towards staff and peers.*

The police were called and I was questioned. What started as going for a walk had escalated beyond all measure of reason. I could have had a police record and lost my ability to work as a teacher. This would have destroyed my career and life as I knew it.

My new risk was that I might make an allegation. The assumption was that what I had to say wasn't true.

The worst part wasn't being restrained, drugged, or suffering an injury. It was being taunted and dehumanised. I tried to hold the student nurse accountable but I was called an aggressor and assaulted. Thankfully, the police saw sense.

I saw how all the violence against me would be justified. In the student nurse's opinion, I wasn't human. Instead, I belonged to a separate species. I felt I had been treated with both prejudice and discrimination. They overlooked so much in order to "treat" my "bad behaviour" quickly that they missed my real issue. They didn't ask questions, and they didn't listen to information which I offered.

The next day I went to OT and spoke to Kathy. My wrist was hurting a lot, and I was upset about what had happened.

01/05/2014 11:27:00 Bone, Kathy

Primrose ward OT notes

Daytime activities

Breakfast club: Alexis approached author on her own volition requesting to be first to cook, reason being she was leaving the ward at 9.30am. Throughout the entire process of cooking bacon, she was noted to be self-directed, methodically working through each step with confidence. Engaged in conversation relating to an incident which occurred earlier in the week stating she had reflected. Although verbally expressed remorse there seemed little remorse in her facial expression. Main focus appeared to be on her own injury therefore dismissing the impact of her behaviour she had on others.

I was remorseful. I still am remorseful! I was sorry Georgia felt scared, if that was what she felt in that moment. I was also flabbergasted that my remorse was questioned. But from an EUPD perspective, I was being emotionally labile. And I was covering my outburst with carefully crafted lies. I was trying to divide and conquer the nursing team.

My facial expressions might not match what I say. I was concerned about my routines, my structures, and predictability. I am concerned with the self. As an autistic woman, I am largely "mind blind". I have taken responsibility for that. I am sorry I didn't express myself in the neurotypical and most socially acceptable way. I'll work on that.

I don't want to be the kind of person who detaches and intellectualises. I was regularly accused of this and staff would insist that I was evading distressing feelings by focusing on logic and information. In fact, I wanted to understand my environment through feelings. I just need a little help to make sense of them.

Such accusations and treatment were very common. It's not stigma around autism or mental illness, but outright discrimination. It's something that as a society we need to overcome. I and the others labelled for the similar behaviours I exhibit are being treated intolerantly in the NHS. And the NHS reflects society.

Many times we have heard about the aggressive autistic boy who shoots his classmates. The fact is, we are not cold aggressors. We do actually have feelings. I have feelings. I might not show them well, but I have them.

*

For a long time, I pondered why Georgia called the police. I feel like a large part of it was because people with neuro-divergence and mental health problems are portrayed as aggressive and unpredictable. This is contrary to evidence that demonstrates we are far more likely to be victims of violence than perpetrators. The narrative portrayed by the media is damaging. Every time autism and mental health is linked to violence, the idea is perpetuated that we are ticking time bombs.

I know I am atypical. For some, my differences are hard to understand. This ambiguity frightens people. Even people like Georgia, who should know better. Since I was seen as the ticking time bomb, she naturally called the police. The staff obviously heard the ridiculous 'I fear for my life' part more clearly than my 'I wanted to go out and she refused to let me, even though I'm informal and it's my legal right.' Oh, and she wound me up by saying, 'You can go out', and then, 'I changed my mind'. She wouldn't have told the police that she laughed and taunted me.

Interestingly, this event wasn't reported to The Retreat to keep me from being accepted to the programme. How curious!

CHAPTER 34

Land's End

We went to Cornwall on a one-week break. I was off section and free from sensory overload. My parents agreed that I could accompany them. The drive from Heysham to Cornwall was long and I counted lamp posts the whole way. White noise created on the fast roads meant the journey was relaxing. Fortunately, Abi is good in the car. She sat pleasantly watching TV on the headrest. We didn't hear a peep out of her.

My parents had rented a three-bedroom house. When we arrived, my mum took us straight to the small, locally owned Cornish pasty shop she always visited. My mum's family are Cornish and she knows the area well. The next few days were quiet and beautiful. I thought how different my experience was compared to the wards and Morecombe Cove. I questioned, only fleetingly, my diseased, mentally-ill brain. Why wasn't it ill now?

We went to St Michael's Mount, a tidal, rocky island crowned with a medieval church and castle. You can walk from the shore to the castle when the tide is out. It's a short walk – even Mum did it. When the tide is in, it's an island. I thought of Alcatraz. Detention was never far from my mind.

We also went to Trengwainton Flower Garden and Land's End. Abi loves flowers. On this day trip, we watched all manner of flowers playing in the sun. The bees buzzed busily between each, and Abi squealed excitedly.

Each evening, after a long day of gentle activity, I played with Abi. We would get a soft foam ball and roll it around in the garden. She was Bambi-like in her movements; clumsy, wobbly, and uncoordinated. The opposite to me. I thought how perfect she was.

Abi most loved to cuddle and roll around the grass. The sun was hot and setting. It was beautiful due to the pollution – smoke particles filter out colours, leaving the vivid pinks, reds, and oranges. Abi and I lay on our backs looking up at the clouds, her body pressed against mine. I told Abi that due to our 300-mile atmosphere, when the sun sets we are lucky to get the scattered light effect. It's because the earth acts as a prism. Predictably, she smiled and kissed me. She didn't know what I was saying but I liked to tell her stuff like that.

I remember being in Land's End when Josh, Thomas, and I were young. It was super-windy. Today was hot and sunny as I thought of Josh being literally blown off his feet. Thomas and I laughed and laughed as he fell face down, while we clung to a gate to avoid the same fate.

Now looking at the exposed cliff edge with its brilliant blue background, I admired the sheer drop to the rocky, granite-ridden waters below, and was struck by the dangerous beauty of the place. The cliffs are spectacular. I calculated that they must have ranged from about 60 to 120 metres high. I took pictures of Abi and worked out the speed I would fall should I jump, and the deceleration speed on the shiny granite rocks. I didn't jump. I wanted to live.

We sat eating Cornish pasties on a bench overlooking the sea. The familiar bite of the Cornish treat was reassuring as I put thoughts of my obsession / fixation from my mind. Right in that moment, I was just enjoying my parents and my daughter. We hadn't sat like that for such a long time. None of us were thinking about doctors, sections, or drugs – the beautiful surroundings distracted us from the reality of the mental health system.

On our last day we all went to Kynance Cove. Located on the west side of the Lizard peninsula, Thomas, Josh, and I used to play there as kids. The coastline is spectacular with picturesque rocks, crystal clear waters, white sands, and caves. We would play hide-and-seek in the caves until high tide when the water reaches the foot of the cliffs. During low tide, we would enjoy the white sand and Thomas and I would build sandcastles while Josh befriended random children. I walked down to the water with Abi waddling beside me, over the cove's white sand beach scattered with dark red and green serpentine rock. We splashed in the water and watched the fish swim in and out of our feet, and went crabbing with a fishing net we bought from the shop.

Holding Abi's hand, I thought, *This is my child. I am a mother. I am not sick or defective.*

CHAPTER 35

York at Last

23rd June 2014

I went to York with HCA Robin and another nurse. Before I left, they gave me two injections to sedate me on the journey. I had lorazepam and olanzapine, and slept most of the way, waking only because I needed to go to the toilet. They didn't want to stop, so I had to hold it for a couple of hours.

When we got there, Robin was like, 'Wow, this is amazing. I wouldn't mind living here.' Robin and I went for a walk around the huge grounds for half an hour just to stretch our legs while the Primrose nurse did the handover. Robin and I were tearful. She gave me a big hug. Robin had truly cared for me for a year and a half.

A nurse named Kim admitted me. She was feisty, with a nose stud, Doc Martin boots, jeans, and a loose top – always her uniform, I came to notice. She looked as though she was going to a rock concert. When Kim finished checking me over physically and asking me questions about my risk, she showed me to my room. She started to leave, and I asked, 'But don't you need some of my stuff?'

'No,' she explained. 'We trust you with it. If you feel unsafe, let us know and we will help you through as a community.

You don't need to hurt yourself with us here.' So, I sat there for the first time, in my room with razors, my belt, skipping rope, and all the other day stuff I usually wasn't allowed, a bit of humanity returned to me.

I was introduced to a client, as distressed people were referred to here, called Kat. She was my buddy. The buddy system helps you settle into the new environment. Kat's parents were both doctors. Kat was quiet, unassuming, and very clever.

Kat helped me through my probation week. In this time, I had to show commitment to the programme, attend all groups, and spend all meals and free time with others in the community. It was easy to do these things because I was eager to do them. It was also easy to sign myself out! I could go into the community just by signing a board and noting what time I'd be back. I didn't have to ask anyone for permission.

Kat was 24 and had been in the system for more than a decade. Like me, she found there was dignity and respect in the Acorn programme. Already, I could feel myself coming back. At the end of probation week, you have to write a letter to the community asking them to accept you into the programme. If they don't, you can't join. I got to the end of the second week. I'd spent hours writing my letter. I read it out in the end-of-week meeting to all the community, including the clients, nurses, HCAs, the doctor, and the psychologist, Philip.

Holly was the first to speak after I read my letter. Everyone else sat quietly, looking at me. Holly had a spiky Mohican. She had a lot of facial piercings and wore blue lipstick. Her arms were like chicken skin where she'd cut so much. She was incredible, really; bright, funny, and talented. She said, 'I've got no idea what you just said, Alexis. I'm sorry, but we don't speak French here. You have to write it again. And when you do, think of other people. We need to be able to understand why you want to be here.'

Everybody else agreed, 'We have no idea what you just said.'

The only person who spoke up for me was a clinical psychologist named Philip. He said, 'I understood it and it was really good. But the community has asked you to do it again, so maybe you can just do it again on Monday. We're not saying you can't be in the programme. We're just saying we don't understand your application.'

I think my letter was too academic and maybe a little verbose. When I wrote the letter, it felt concise. I had consulted several academic texts. That was apparently where I went wrong. I wasn't getting in touch with my "feelings". But I didn't know my feelings then.

This was the first time I had an overload and a meltdown in Acorn. I walked, disorientated, along the side of Heslington Road, the main road The Retreat was on. I lost my sense of balance and was likely twirling. A police car stopped. They asked me questions, but I couldn't respond.

York has an open-door policy. Staff and clients must sit with the anxiety of somebody walking out. Community rules are that clients cannot be prevented from leaving or from self-harming. Even in an extreme case, if somebody says 'I'm going to go kill myself. You can all fuck off,' and they leave, you're not allowed to go after them. If more than two people in the community believe it's a credible threat, then you can phone the police, but you're not allowed to go after them yourself.

I wasn't aware that Holly and another client, Diane, had come after me. They were present when the police handcuffed me, put me in their caged car and took me back. I was told it was the first time this sort of incident had happened in The Retreat. Holly and Diane were notably shocked, as was I. They had to justify coming after me, saying it was because they were so taken aback at my presentation. It wasn't a personality disorder presentation.

Philip had the information about my suspected autism from Primrose's psychologists, Reggine and Felicity. The clients didn't get that information. Philip probably hadn't read it by then either, since I'd only been there for a few days.

I was asked by the community to complete what they called a behaviour analysis. It was useful to track how everything unfolded, but I already knew. Something unexpected happens, my head feels like it will explode, and then it does. The analysis is a two-page document that you have to read out. It's embarrassing but not punishment.

Interestingly, I didn't kick off. I guess that's because the doors were open and I wasn't feeling physically constrained. The police stopped to help, worried about my lack of balance and unresponsiveness. I wasn't doing anything dangerous. If they had known of autism, then perhaps they wouldn't have stopped. Perhaps I would have been free to express myself in a way that suits me.

When the police got involved there was still no kick-off. It was more like my brain had shut down. It wasn't allowing more information in. The doors were open. I was free and moving. I learnt quickly that after 45 minutes of movement, I can be fine again. This was an important discovery. I could also calm myself using the techniques Reggine had given me. I could manage my behaviour myself. I didn't need others to manage it for me.

The Retreat was proactive. It was calm. The boundaries gave structure, and you could listen and be listened to within the structure. Clients and staff tried to help sort problems out before they even became a nuisance, let alone an issue and certainly not an incident. I spent most of my time outside gardening and joined a leisure centre and spa club.

I met Bex, who is now a lifelong friend. She is a doctor and triathlete. Bex was at Edinburgh University at the same time that I was. She had a diagnosis of personality disorder and an eating disorder. I didn't notice them. Bex was very exacting and quite withdrawn. She was very shy and would curl her five-foot frame into the smallest ball in an armchair. We got along great.

I was Bex's buddy to help her settle into the programme. Our friendship grew from that. She's the first real friend I've had who can relate to every aspect of me.

Sometimes it's easier to be friends, or at least talk with people, who also have mental health problems. You are not judged but understood. This is what it was like for Bex and me. After every group, we would go for a walk and talk through what had just happened. Bex helped me to understand how others were feeling, and I encouraged her to speak more. In the mornings, we would go for a run. I never got lost despite my poor cognitive map because Bex was a human GPS system. We didn't talk much during runs. We just felt the freedom and enjoyed the companionship.

Bex would notice when I was getting overloaded and would let me know in the nicest and kindest of ways. Together, we would sit in the sensory room and relax for a while. The room was specially designed combining a range of stimuli like lights, colours, sounds, and sensory soft play objects, all within a safe environment. I loved using it to explore and interact. There was no risk – it was calming.

I was getting all the sensory feedback and space I needed. The filled-up balloon of my head was now half empty. Abi's toys were not flashing or making noise in my space, and my mum was not worrying because I'd walked out the door. It was the best I'd been in a year and a half. I just knew that I would get better here. There was so much hope. This was it.

I was finally eating a balanced diet again. Every meal, I had three or four options. I always went to the post-meal support group. Here we talked about our dinner experience. Bex went because she struggled with food. When asked about how she found dinner, she always said, 'Fine'. This aggravated the community. I didn't know what else they wanted her to say. I went because I found the smells and noise of people eating difficult. We both needed a break after dinner and post-meal support group, so we would play catch on the ginormous lawn outside our mansion home.

I had a voice. I was involved in my treatment, and I was responsible for others. In this community, everyone had responsibilities that rotated weekly. These were not the meaningless jobs I had in acute wards or PICUs. At the start of each week we would meet, with a woman chairperson to run the group. One person had to shop for the community, because on the weekend we cooked for ourselves. Somebody else would manage the budget and get money from the finance office.

We all had influence, and we had control over how we lived and ran our community. These were the keys to my feeling so great. Formal and informal barriers were removed. This powerfully transformed relations between clients and staff. We were, at least superficially, all equal. There were lots of opportunities in the hospital for clients. For example, you could be on the panel to interview prospective newcomers.

I read up on my counselling skills and created a scheme of work to train peer support workers. I got to use my skills as a teacher. I delivered groups in the Acorn programme and learnt about inspections for the Care Quality Commission. I went down to a conference in London, learning the criteria for accrediting therapeutic communities. This was the first time I used my experiences as a distressed person to do something productive. Bex was too shy to do much of this, but she supported me in it.

I felt so good that something productive was coming from the suffering I had experienced. I spoke to new nurses and was involved in staff training. I could be worthwhile.

I would leave this place to go home.

My hope continued to grow for about two months. Previously, I was having meltdowns every other day and they were bad, with restraints and injections. Now the medication which masked my pain and distress was being gradually reduced. I was dealing with things on my own. By the time I left,

I was nearly off all my medication except Ritalin. I needed that drug to sit through all the groups and actually concentrate.

The problem with overload, though, never went away. Every three or four weeks, there would be an incident. As the weeks went on, the difference between me and the rest of the community became more pronounced. It was causing difficulty. Bex was the only person I could relate to. The community also didn't like that we were such good friends. They would say we had an exclusive relationship. This wasn't the case. We would invite them on walks, runs, and to go to the gym but only Kat ever wanted to join us.

Because of the self-defeating behaviours of the group, in the mornings you'd hear, 'I feel really shit, I want to cut myself, I hate my life, everything is crap, I just want to die.' We'd go around the circle and you'd hear it from every single person, except Bex who always said she was, 'Fine'. It made no sense to me. I felt sad, like I'm sorry you feel that way. I didn't understand the emotions these women felt and I couldn't understand or rationalise the intensity with which they felt them.

I tried my best to understand and was active in the groups. I wanted to be helpful. I was rational and these women were emotional. I thought I could cut through their emotions and make them see how irrational their thoughts were, and this would help. So, I would copy what the nurses or Phillip, the psychologist, would say. Then I mirrored it. This was encouraged. Each person was seen as a therapist / support for others.

There was an average of four hours of DBT-focused groups per day. During the morning DBT groups, clients would talk about what they called "urges". I had no urges at all. They all had high urges. Bex had urges to let blood. She wanted to cut her artery and bleed as much as possible until she needed a transfusion. I understood how it could make her feel better, and I supported her in not doing it. When she felt bad, we would run. It worked every time. We were both doing great. We were good for each other.

Each week we had a card with five urges that we felt on it. Each day we had to score the strength of the urge from 1 to 10. But I had no urges. My nurse said, 'Write what you do have, what is difficult.'

The only thing I had the urge to do was move. But it wasn't an urge. It was stronger than that, like a compulsion. If I didn't do it, I wasn't regulated. Was the fleeing I did when things were too much an urge? I didn't think so. It just happened. It was fight or flight. Was it an urge that I wanted to get away from intense sound?

I still had blank boxes on my DBT card. This set me apart from the others. Bex tried to explain the card but I couldn't understand the format. I said, 'You just can't reduce behaviour to a number.' I told staff I had conducted some research as part of my Masters in Education and behaviour is not an urge. So, what do I do? Argh, I just couldn't understand. It worked for others, but not for me. I felt weird again. But it was a small issue, right?

It was agreed that for me the numbers would change to red, green, and yellow. Instead of urges, I would choose a DBT skill and try to master it. If I did well the square would go green. Because my DBT card was different, the rest of the community was unhappy. 'Oh, you're being treated differently.' As a community that ran ourselves, the women made it an issue. The staff rarely override discussion or close the case, so to speak.

Other clients didn't seem to respond quickly to environment, therapy, and DBT skills as I did. They were constantly consumed with thoughts of harming. Even with the therapy and talk time available, they struggled. I couldn't help but think, *You're in this beautiful environment and you still want to hurt yourself?* Even when we had just discussed a good DBT skill like "opposite to emotion-action", they didn't use the skill. I would tell them, 'Okay, so you feel like you want to go to bed. Use the opposite action to the emotion. So, that would mean going for a walk instead of going to bed.' But no, they still hurt. I learnt a lot from them about emotions. Their emotions were so visible and this helped me to see mine a little clearer.

Bex would always talk through with me why people acted the way they did. But my ability to understand what they might be thinking didn't improve. Sometimes I might say an inappropriate thing, when I'd let my mind go and hadn't masked or mirrored. Then there would be this awful silence. This gap between me and the group continued to widen.

I had a DBT intervention once a week with my named nurse, Scott. I booked a time and it always happened then. This was wonderful. I had to book it a week in advance at least, so all the ownership was on me. In that meeting, with no urges to discuss, we focused on DBT strategies. We were doing emotional regulation.

The first skill involved recognising and naming emotions. It was the first time I had been challenged to do this. Suddenly I couldn't fake it till I made it!

Scott was patient with me. Anxiety and anger were the first emotions I identified. We used descriptive labels such as "frustrated" or "anxious" rather than what I said before, such as 'I feel full up' or 'My brain feels like it's about to explode'. However, over the coming months, these descriptors never transferred into actual feelings. Scott and I realised they were two separate things.

Scott had a sheet of words associated with depression. Meaninglessness and hopelessness were under depression. So, I realised that although I wasn't depressed, I had characteristics which related to that.

In DBT class, we were also given an acronym: PLEASE MASTER. The advice this acronym gave was to help reduce emotional vulnerability:

PL – represents taking care of our physical health.

E – is for eating a balanced diet and avoiding excess sugar, fat, and caffeine.

A – stands for avoiding alcohol and drugs, or anything which increases emotional instability.

S – represents getting a good sleep.

E – is for exercise.

MASTER – refers to doing daily activities that build confidence and competency.

We were told that we would be working on this for some time. I looked at it and thought, *I do all these anyway.*

And also, I'm not emotionally vulnerable. I don't feel emotions so they don't make me vulnerable. This didn't go down at all well with the group, who needed to work on a lot of the above. The homework set each week was all like this. Again, the gap between me and others widened.

Phillip, the psychologist, said, 'We think you have alexithymia.' I thought, *Great, something else to add to the list.* Thankfully in York, they don't work with diagnosis. That's why it's called a programme for women with self-defeating behaviour. They work with the underlying causes of behaviour, rather than a "we're going to fix you" approach.

I understood the emotional regulation topic. I learnt all the skills and memorised them. I couldn't relate to the emotions but I could recall the skills by rote. For the other clients, this topic was essential. One minute they'd be fine, and the next they'd be displaying very distressing behaviour.

Dysregulation was frowned upon because there is a lot of opportunity to manage it. In an acute unit they would have been upturning tables. You could see emotion fizzing under their skin, but it rarely escaped because of the support. Maybe only once every three weeks somebody might shout. The community would hold the person to account by exploring, using a behavioural analysis, why it happened. Like, 'Why didn't you use this skill?' or 'You need to practice that skill more'. Bex was the opposite of the others. She would say she was "Fine", when sometimes she wasn't. She was impossible for them to read and that set her apart. Bex talked to me, though, so I always knew what was going on with her.

Every couple of weeks, I would have an overload. I wouldn't be able to speak or respond. I would go for a walk with Bex. That always helped. The community was getting sick of my lack of progress. Bex could see my improvement when no one else could. She knew how hard I was trying. They said, 'You're doing the same behaviour over and over and you're not learning from it. You're not using DBT.' The unacceptable behaviour trigger was sensory overload.

Even Scott would ask, 'What progress have you made? You did that in week one and we're now in month two ... month three ... month four.'

In an overload, the only way I could communicate was on a whiteboard. I'd go into the sensory room and interact with objects in this unrestrained, non-threatening space. When I was ready, I would write everything on the whiteboard. The community didn't understand this.

Weeks passed. Jobs in the community rotated and I became the person responsible for shopping. Things had settled down. I was fine. But I still had overload from all the information I was learning. My balloon was still half full. I was nervous about the shop and the trip because the community was counting on me. I had a lot to remember. It was stressful to shop for myself, let alone for 10 other people.

When I walked into the supermarket, I had already done a full day of therapy. My balloon was full. I was like, *Whoa!* The strips of lights that run down the aisles were so bright, as if I was on a runway. When I looked at the shelves, patterns and numbers jumped out at me in 3D. It was like the numbers were removed from the packaging. The way things moved was blurry as though they were going fast. Certain things popped out, like when I looked at a trolley, I would see all the squares in the metal. I realised it was impossible for me to do the shopping for the community.

I fed back my experience to the group in the morning meeting. When it was my turn I said, 'That was odd,' about the shopping. I told them my experience. Instead of the usual feedback, I got nothing. I don't think they knew what to say. I felt weird. This was happening a lot. Being open isn't so bad when people share the same experiences as you, but this was not okay.

Then the next person would say, 'I want to die.'

The next woman would say, 'I just wanted to make myself sick all night.'

Then Bex would say, 'I'm fine.'

It was clear that I didn't feel like them, and they didn't share anything I felt. It was as if I was in the wrong place. I could never respond emotionally to them. I tried. I did the mirroring like, 'You must've been very angry about that.' For them, it was a relief to talk about their feelings. For me, it was bloody hard work.

When I went into the group, I knew I had a whole hour of having to think about my tone, my voice intonation, the way I was sitting, and my stimming. I used to tic quite a bit. It was how I coped, also a response to certain meds. This didn't go down well. I would be working hard to respond, like counselling for an hour. I had to deploy loads of social skills. I would be knackered by the end of it. It was a cognitive overload. My brain was full trying to manage this new workload, coupled with the fact I was doing something I just didn't understand. Then I would walk or run in complete silence through the beautiful hospital grounds and all was well with the world.

*

Basically, the motto was, if you have a secret then you have a problem. Everything was to be shared with the group. Our only one-on-one therapy was for an hour a week with the psychologist Mark. I wanted to talk to him about Josh. I felt I was in the right place. However, until your behaviour was stable you couldn't do trauma work.

Most of these girls had horrific back stories, like sexual abuse. One lady had been in the war in Iraq. Whenever a helicopter flew overhead, she would dive onto the floor. Until you can manage emotions and refrain from self-defeating behaviours like the cutting, ligaturing, the fluid restriction, there is no trauma work. The work is learning DBT skills and then using them to keep safe.

For me, I was stable, but my problem, according to them, was that I couldn't learn from my mistakes. The overloads were my "mistakes". I could see why they would think this, and this was the source of my downfall. I agreed with them. When 10 people are suggesting you aren't doing enough and you aren't learning, you tend to believe them. So, I thought, too, *I'm just not trying hard enough.*

We practised DBT every day in groups, meetings, at lunch and dinner, and I read up afterwards from the workbook. I knew every sentence. I could tell you where the sentence was on which page because I could see the patterns of letters and I loved numbers. But I just wasn't applying the skills, was I?

CHAPTER 36

Diagnosis – High-Functioning Autism

I was about to get lucky again. I didn't know it, and I didn't feel lucky.

As weeks went by, I tried harder to fit in by "feeling" things. I was getting overwhelmed and full up trying to process. One day, I had a meltdown. I left The Retreat and just ran. I was inside myself, unaware of my surroundings. It was dark and I ran through the streets of York. I found my way back to The Retreat some 45 minutes later. I was calmer but unable to vocalise much of anything I was feeling. I was drawing on the board in the sensory room trying to explain to an HCA. I was counting and moving in circles. The HCA called the on-call doctor. This happened to be Dr Alyssa Barton, the lead doctor specialising in autism in the hospital. I was so, so lucky. If I hadn't had a meltdown on that day, at that time, I might never have known what was different about me.

From the notes I read later, I was walking in circles in the sensory room, counting and clicking. Dr Barton, the on-call doctor, sat in the room discreetly watching. After about 45 minutes, she quietly moved closer, knelt down, and said, 'Would you like to use the weighted blanket?' She put the weighted blanket on me, and after a while she asked, 'Would you like to use the fibre-optic cables?' They're long, 10-metre cables, like a horse's tail. They're wonderful because they gently change colour. They're tactile, visual, and very soothing. She turned those on. I calmed down. Later, when I was oriented, she put a projector on. That freaked me out so she turned it off.

I just sat with the blanket and the cables, and she sat with me. When everything was fine, she left. The next day she came to see me. She introduced herself and asked, 'Do you remember me?'

I said, 'I remember somebody, but I don't look at people's faces really.'

She said, 'My name is Dr Alyssa Barton.' She explained that she had spoken to my team. She strongly believed I was autistic, and that I'd had a meltdown. She said she wanted to do more testing with me.

When she told me, I was like, 'I'm a teacher. I've taught kids with autism, and I'm definitely not autistic.' But after some days in which Bex and I read up on autism and looked at the different ways it manifests, it seemed plausible. Bex reassured me and I trusted her as she was a doctor and I knew she looked at me objectively. She was good at making clinical decisions. She was also humane. I didn't want to leave York, so I was hesitant about doing the test. But later my mum and I agreed that I should.

My mum drove up from Morecombe Cove and I did a five-hour interview with Dr Barton. Two weeks later, I did one with Dr Liz Hadley, a clinical psychologist from The Tuke Centre which is part of The Retreat. Dr Hadley initially thought I was drunk as I had such bad sensory overload that I was wobbly as I walked up the stairs to her office. I reassured her that I didn't drink. When we got to the end, I was fatigued. It was taxing doing test after test. It's a very intense diagnostic process.

After the assessment, Dr Hadley sat down with me. I was having some water because I was thirsty after all the tests. She showed me the results, and said, 'Alexis, I want to let you know that you're not ill.'

I was so overwhelmed. I said, 'What is it then?'

She said, 'You have high-functioning autism.' At that point I vomited into the cup I was holding. I felt nothing but overwhelmed.

She said, 'You're not mentally ill. You are autistic.'

After almost two years of hellish "treatment", here's the doctor telling me I'm not ill. Her report explained my seemingly odd behaviour. My behaviour now seemed to have a context and wasn't so odd. Over time, Dr Hadley gave a framework to understand my experiences and I knew in that moment that I would be forever grateful to her.

I didn't have a personality disorder. The Retreat gave me the space to figure all this out. I could see that therapy had its limits to helping my difference. Now we knew why. Bex always said that I was a therapy expert, but that its effects were negligible on me. It was sad when I realised this too. I thought I was finally on the mend.

When I have a meltdown, I flee. This happened again in October 2014. I learnt that fleeing is very common for autistics. I ran into York City Centre, 1.4 miles from The Retreat. There is an abundance of police all over York. It feels like they're at every corner because it's a big city for England. The police caught me. By this time, we'd had a meeting with the police liaison, so they knew not to touch me. These were plain clothes officers. By now I was traumatised by uniforms. I couldn't calm down. This had been building for a few weeks. They had to put me in a cage to take me to the 136 suite, a place where people who are sectioned under the Section 136 of the Mental Health Act are taken. The Retreat isn't considered a place of safety for me because there are no locked doors.

Slowly in the 136 suite, I came back. Then I felt sad. I knew I was in trouble with the other clients. I hadn't tried hard enough again. What was wrong with me? The ward manager came to see me and so did Dr Barton. They drove me back to The Retreat in their car.

Now I was on a Section 2 of the Mental Health Act, for assessment. Remember I had to be voluntary (off section) to go to Acorn, so now I was officially fucked!

When I went back, I didn't go into any groups to start with. I didn't want to face people and listen to them telling me how I hadn't tried. Bex would come in my room and sit with me for hours. And I had Roo, the cuddly baby kangaroo from *Winnie the Pooh* which I bought for Abi when she came for her next visit. Bex would sit with Roo on her lap and talk. We would play backgammon and Scrabble. I usually won Scrabble, but she was getting good at backgammon.

After two or three days, I was able to attend groups. They helped, actually. I applied DBT skills to manage my feelings. I still wasn't able to tag many emotions. I was restless, couldn't concentrate, and found conversation hard.

I was obsessed with suicide and hanging. I had to read about it six times a day. I was also frequently tying nooses when staff were not looking. It's hard to describe why I had to do it. You know if you "need" the toilet, you just have to go. This was the same kind of feeling.

If you're put on a section in The Retreat you have to leave on what's called a timeout. This is supposed to provide space for you and the community to reflect, evaluate, and decide the best way forward. Bex thought I didn't need space. She thought I just needed to figure out how to reduce overloads. She said this to the group, the only time I had heard her speak up, but they shot her down. *Great way to encourage her to open up,* I thought.

I was given work to do. I had to reflect on what had happened. I had to write a statement saying how I would devise management strategies so I wouldn't melt down again.

Even thinking of this homework now, I realise how different my "issue" and "behaviour" was to other people's. I couldn't even think of how I might go about this. There are university professors and autism experts trying to devise these very things every day with limited success.

The community decided I needed the timeout. I had to go. I couldn't go home because I was sectioned, so my only option was to go to an acute unit. I knew this would make me worse and start the whole cycle of admissions again. Bex was afraid for me. She agreed to call me every day and she did. That was a lot for her because she never calls anyone.

My worry about the transfer increased and so did my compulsion. Bex and I spent longer together, if that was possible. I didn't want to leave her, my best friend. We were good for each other. On 4th November, I was transferred by secure ambulance to Blackthorn hospital in Heysham. I was told I could come back when I was not in a "crisis". I gave Bex Abi's Roo. I figured she needed it more than Abi.

CHAPTER 37

Desperate

4th November 2014

I didn't want to go. I didn't want to leave.

York staff prepared me well. I knew in the morning I would be going to Clover Ward that night. I was furious about this. I had made an advanced directive with Kim on the day I arrived in York that should I be sectioned again and receive forced treatment I wouldn't be readmitted to Clover. Any ward except Clover.

In Clover, the corridors were narrow and had no natural light. The ceiling was lined with bright lights. The old asylum acoustics were a challenge because noise travelled. And there was no courtyard, nowhere to run. All these disturbances made my job of proving I was suitable to return to The Retreat much more difficult. It was feeling impossible, really. I tried to reason with the doctor and the manager of The Retreat to no avail.

*

It was late evening. I was waiting for the ambulance to come. I said goodbye to Bex.

Scott brought a social worker along to accompany me. Scott said, 'You have to go now. It's time, Alexis.' Bex left for a run. We had agreed on that.

Unable to come to terms with what was happening, I said, 'I'm not going.' Sending me away was a mistake. I knew I could get better here, whatever better looked like. I had no chance in Clover. I knew the triggers now. I knew what overloaded me. I pleaded and tried to reason with them, but they wouldn't engage. Still I refused to leave. I wanted to protest how unfair this transfer was.

Three huge men, and I mean big, bigger than me, came into my room. They took my arms and feet and gently "encouraged" me to the car. I say encouraged because it wasn't abusive like a restraint. They didn't hurt me. My skin was uncomfortable but not on fire since I was more settled. I wasn't screaming in pain and pulling away.

It was the most humane transfer I'd ever had. A huge minivan was there, like a normal car with the windows blacked out. It was brand new and nice. I hadn't seen guys like these. They were like huge bouncers and super-muscly. If it had been any other time, I would've said, 'Hello, boys!'

I didn't have a meltdown but I was so desperate. I struggled to not get into the car. York was the place where I was certain that afterwards I would go home. I was in such a state. They were restraining me much of the way. Slowly I calmed down. My stubbornness, not wanting to accept my fate, came out.

I must say that was first time I was deliberately obstructive. I knew going back to Heysham I would be treated like shit. They had contacted PICU. They had already decided I was a disastrous nightmare. Staff were heavy-handed and uncaring, and they knew I couldn't manage acute. They knew it and they planned for it.

The day before my arrival I saw in the notes that the Out of Hours management plan for me was:

OOHs Clinical Lead

c/o admission. Agreed the following management plan in consultation with Paola Walters and Robin Fields:

1) *Oaken and Primrose moved PSTS trained staff to Clover who will have a total of four PSTS trained staff on duty nocte*

2) *Staffing level increased to six nocte*

3) *Contact duty dr c/o pharmacological intervention on arrival*

4) *Chase up PICU referral 5/11/14*

5) *All wards are alerted to attend Clover ASAP when blicks* [alarms staff wear on their belts] *go off*

The ambulance pulled in. Four staff, all men, were waiting at the door. They were ready to pounce on me. Scared, I tried to flee. They grabbed me and wrestled me into the ward. 'For fuck's sake,' I screamed. I hadn't been treated like this for five months!

They let me go. I was shaken but calm. *Great, thank you.* I could see I was in for more restraint and injections.

I managed, though. I completed all the work I was given. I used my new DBT skills to minimise sensory overload and meltdown. Mostly I used interpersonal effectiveness. This provided a template to talk to staff. I could finally attend to relationships and build a sense of mastery in socialising. I used the lesson where I had learnt to articulate what I wanted from an interaction. I could not do this prior to York. That's why I had so many problems. But now I knew what I needed to do to get the results I wanted.

The name of the specific skill I used was **DEAR MAN.**

Describe the current situation

Express your feelings and opinions

Assert yourself by asking for what you want, or by saying no

Reward the person – let them know what they will get out of it

Mindful of objectives without distraction (broken record technique, ignoring attacks)

Appear effective and competent (role play, use your acting skills)

Negotiate alternative solutions

I was so glad I had learnt this. I thought how useful DBT was for the general populace, not just those in distress. I had fewer social issues and confusions on the ward. I could talk to staff. I just had to prepare my **DEAR MAN.** My success rate for needs being met went up.

I was desperate to get back to York to learn more. I was told often that I would be going back soon. I was constantly in contact with the nurses there. Bex said the clients were updated on my progress every day. Also, staff in Clover were in contact with the Acorn Unit. See from my hospital clinical notes below:

Contacted Acorn Unit and spoke with deputy manager and Miss Quinn's named nurse Scott who informed that there is a time out agreement created for Alexis and she can return to Acorn if she complies with this agreement for the next 14 days. Informed Dr O about the plan and a professionals meeting arranged on Friday 7th.

*

The daily phone contact with The Retreat helped me feel like I was still part of the programme. But it was easy to get dejected. My new skills meant I could talk this feeling through, though. This helped so much.

I was expressing myself and articulating difficulties. Armed with an autism diagnosis there was some understanding from staff. Not much, I have to say. But I wasn't treated like an attention seeker when I needed to do certain things. This meant nurses could help me, especially when Reggine got more specific about my autistic needs.

I saw Reggine on the 5th November. We made a plan together that focused on all my autism behaviours that got me in trouble with staff. I had ways now to stay clear on my emotional and physical needs to avoid meltdowns.

I did everything I was asked. Yes, I looked like a weirdo twirling, jumping, and pushing against walls. But I wasn't called names by the staff or told to stop. They saw this "behaviour" positively for once. Felicity, Luke, and especially Reggine helped me understand my new diagnosis.

On 10th November, I went to tribunal. Everyone was assembled but before it started the responsible clinician took me off section. Now I was sure I was going back to The Retreat. I had managed. I had done all my work and faxed proof to The Retreat. I had communicated with them daily as requested.

I thought I would be going back that day or the day after.

I went out on leave with my family. It was nice to be close to home again and see them. Abi was growing fast. She was chatting away and interested in everything. I loved playing with her. However, I was still keen to get back to York to finish the work I had started so I could ensure I had a future.

I spoke to the ward manager on my return from leave. He had just talked to Scott:

Contact received from Scott, Deputy Ward Manager at the Acorn Unit. Scott informed that Alexis needs to have time out for full 14 days. They need this time to do the briefing to other residents. Scott agreed that Alexis can return to Acorn on Wednesday 19th. Scott also informed that she spoke to Wilma the care coordinator and agreed to make referrals to specialist place for autism. Alexis returned to ward around 5.00pm, she asked to speak to the writer and ask for any update regarding her return to Acorn. Writer informed Alexis that a transfer is agreed for 19th and advised her the details of conversation with Scott.

For some reason, The Retreat decided I had to wait until 19th November. I had to do the full 14 days. I was very upset. This felt like punishment to me. What benefit to anybody was that decision? I had done everything they asked of me. The ward was hard work. I had struggled to maintain myself and not get overloaded.

On 15th November, I received a phone call from The Retreat. They said they wouldn't have me back because I was autistic and the mode of therapy they offered was not helpful to me.

One of our major concerns, is your client's real inability to understand the impact her behaviours have had on the Community and while none of us see this as her fault, it severely limits the work we can do with her following what happened. We do feel very strongly that a referral to Falton Green as a specialist service for autism, is the next step for your client. I hope you received the email containing our referral letter to Falton Green as well as the full report of your client's diagnosis.

I was told this by Phillip, the psychologist, over the phone. I had no support on receiving this news. I melted down badly. I thought my life was over. It wouldn't have been so bad if I hadn't been groomed into trusting the staff in York, believing in the therapeutic process and the "community" – where everyone had a say. Bex had no idea this decision had been made, and neither did the clients. So much for their flattened hierarchy. I had trusted them when they said I would come back. Now I felt betrayed and rejected.

*

A referral was made to Falton Green. I now knew that everyone, including the amazing Retreat, thought I needed to go there. I agreed to an assessment. Herbert Ledstone, general manager of the Falton Green unit came to assess me. He sounded positive. This softened the blow.

I was in Clover for six weeks. I didn't hear from Bex much after the decision was made for me not to return. We both cried when I told her. The news was too much for her. After only two weeks, she blood-let and was sent back home on timeout. She wasn't allowed back to The Retreat either. I missed her so much.

I was discharged just before Christmas. I went home with no management plan. I was fine at home for a short time. I had strategies and used them well. It took a good few weeks for my overload to get to a critical level. With no support in the community it was hard to manage.

I had a start date for Falton Green on 29th December. I wasn't sure about attending Falton Green until I had seen it. They didn't have very favourable Care Quality Commission reports. I wanted to check it out.

CHAPTER 38

Spoon Theory

2nd December 2014

While waiting for the Falton Green placement, I identified what causes me to derail. Using the internet, I began to understand my eccentricities. Christine Miserandino's[2] spoon theory helped me clarify my relationship to different kinds of stimuli Miserandino describes how we all have a personal energy level, which she represents as a quantity of spoons. When we do activities, our energy spoons are used up.

On an average day in my normal life, I begin with my 20-spoon supply. Everything's fine, input is modulated, I'm relaxed. I have breakfast with my daughter and she makes loads of noise. This costs me a spoon.

Then I go to school and use up 10 spoons. Class transitions are planned, so they don't take too much energy. I have free periods, scheduled breaks and lunches that provide a rest to replenish some spoons. I get home and Abi's happy to see me and wants interaction. This uses up more spoons. I get to the end of the day and I might have two or three spoons left and it's cool. I use social media. That uses a spoon or two. It's fine. I'm depleted, but it's time for bed.

When my carefully managed life suddenly had unexpected demands, I quickly ran out of spoons. In my life before, if I had an unexpected change I could still manage because I would cut out having lunch with colleagues, or I'd skip dinner to get some quiet time. But as a mother, I couldn't cut out essential activities.

So, for the next three weeks at home I worked on myself. I evaluated my activities. Running in the morning helped. But having an hour-long catch-up with friends depleted spoons. I realised that my emotional, language, and social spoons are like gold. If I used them up early in the day, it was game over for many other things. I had to be smarter in structuring my time.

I mapped what my daily spoon distribution looked like:

Social – three spoons

Language – three spoons

Physical – three spoons

Sensory – five spoons

Executive functioning – six spoons.

I learnt to conserve spoons. It's not good to get to a point where you can't talk. When I had stretched my language and social spoons thinly, I avoided situations guaranteed to use them. I was looking forward to talking with Falton Green about this and seeing what else I could do to improve.

I now identified as an autistic. I no longer felt alone in my struggles. There was this online community, and I learnt from them.

Reading more, I realised why some days I could manage and other days I just couldn't. The autistics in the blogs spoke about how they were always expected to manage. I was familiar with this expectation. Because I could do something one day, I must be able to do it another day. There's pressure for us to always perform, especially if considered smart. They called it ableism.

When I had lost my ordered life, I didn't know what the hell was going on. That was difficult enough, leading to the first hospitalisation. Then going into an absolutely chaotic environment with zero predictability and structure – it was impossible. I don't know how I lasted. Well, I nearly didn't last.

CHAPTER 39

Autism Specialist Unit

30th December 2014

Straight away funding was approved by the Out of Area Treatment panel. Out of Area Treatment (OATs) panels meet to decide who gets to have the treatment they need and where they receive that treatment if it cannot be provided locally. What was in the pot for The Retreat was transferred to Falton Green Therapeutic Campus.

My parents and I made the three-hour drive to take a look. Falton Green was its own small village surrounded by village homes. Each unit was a large house with a garden. A roundabout was in the centre of the village.

I had researched the place. The area was quiet and sleepy. However, I was worried a little by the numerous newspaper articles I read asserting that patients could be heard distressed – screaming, shouting to the extent that neighbours had set up a noise monitoring system. Apparently, residents were locked inside and had been seen banging their heads on the windows. Obviously, this was alarming to me. Even the neighbours exclaimed that the patients needed help and that Falton Green obviously wasn't the right place for them.

When I arrived, I was greeted warmly by Herbert Ledstone, the manager. Also joining the look-around was Alejandro, a psychologist. Falton Green seemed fine, in a beautiful rural area. The running would be picturesque. I could see myself there, surrounded by fields and learning about autism.

So, I agreed to go. A date was set for my admission, 29th December 2014. My brother Thomas drove me. We had dinner on the way at a nice restaurant. Thomas wasn't easy about the place on arrival because we were met by an HCA who presented as uncaring. She seemed to view me as an inconvenience. Thomas felt this and said, 'Are you sure, Lex?'

Well, I had weighed up all my options.

I was free in the sense that I wasn't on section. However, you are only allowed to stay in the community if you abide by the rules. This includes adhering to the authorities' ideas of treatment.

I knew, at present, I couldn't function in the community. I didn't know why. And the special interest in suicide? Autism? I thought this would be a chance to learn and figure things out.

I said to Thomas, 'Yes, I'm sure. Hopefully I'll be home in a couple of months.' The staff had suggested a three-month assessment with occupational therapy and psychology. I needed the psychology to process Josh's death. I hadn't been able to speak of it.

The HCA Heidi took me to the female unit. Thomas left. He didn't see the inside. If he had, I know he would've taken me home. But it was too late.

As I walked in the door, the airlock slammed behind me. From the outside the place looked nice. Inside, it stank. Later I realised it had never been so clean as when I had the tour. When they knew I was coming, they must have scrubbed.

Now there was sick all over the floor. I came to know the three-times-a-day puker as Fiona. She had been a hairdresser. She was a loud, gregarious, and funny lady.

Fiona didn't like to put on weight. She was labelled as anorexic. But the way she described the purging as a compulsive act, it seemed part of her autism. Fiona was a smoker. If she didn't purge within 20 minutes of eating, staff rewarded her with a "treat cigarette". She would comply with this request, but not much else.

Dirt was everywhere. The unit is supposed to be cleaned by its residents. Obviously, they didn't much feel like cleaning. It looked like it hadn't been vacuumed for months. It was a tiny house. This was homey when I first visited. Two people my size would brush shoulders if they passed one another in the corridor. Now it was a claustrophobic, smelly, and intense place.

I noticed for the first time the heavy hospital doors. These were a step up in security. It was a locked ward, more secure than an acute ward and almost the same as PICU.

Reassured by being informal, I decided I needed to go for a run to see the fields. I dropped my stuff in my huge room on a private wing of the first floor. I shared the wing with one other girl on a Section 37/41, a court order. This means she had committed a criminal offence but hadn't gone to prison. She was alright, not aggressive. We had our own TV room up there. There was a door with a key code that separated it from the other rooms.

I was put on a 1:1 with a very young HCA called Misty. This immediately irritated me. I didn't need someone watching me. I was informal. I said to her, 'I want to go out for a jog.'

She said, 'No, you can't go out.'

'What do you mean, I can't go out? I'm informal. It's law that I can go out.' Misty shrugged. She explained it wasn't her decision. I knew that already. I know the system.

The nurses' office was downstairs. I went through the three locked upstairs doors and ran down the stairs. I knocked on the door. After some time, it opened. I walked in and a hand stopped me. Ah, yes. I remembered patients may not share the same space as staff. I stepped back.

The nurse, Taisha, was a black woman as tall as me. She said, 'You can't go out for 72 hours.'

I'm like, 'I can. You can't do that. I know the law. As an Informal patient if I ask to go out, unless you put me on a Section 5(4) or Section 5(2), you can't stop me. So, unless you're going to do that, you need to let me out.' Well, it was a big mistake saying that.

Taisha says, 'I'm going to call the doctor. She will decide whether to put you on a Section 5(2).'

'I'm sorry, but while you're calling the doctor, I'm going out for a jog.'

'Well, no, you're not.'

'Yes, I am.'

She went back in the office. My heart was beating fast. I looked around. Only an hour ago I was driving here with my brother, full of hope. I stood looking at the small corridor filled with the heavy smell of sick, and wails from other patients. I panicked.

Impulsively, I grabbed HCA Misty's lanyard with the fob to open the front airlock door. I opened the first door, opened the second. I ran out of the cul-de-sac that was Falton Green.

I'm autistic. I didn't think about what the staff would be thinking. My only concern was that I wanted a run. I'm informal and legally entitled to run when I want, within reason. I had no thought about what Falton Green's response would be.

I didn't know the area so I assumed if I went right, right, and right, I'd come back to the hospital. Off I jogged and turned right. I ran for about a mile. I thought to myself, *Gosh, this is a long road.* Suddenly a blue car, a large, old Ford Focus Estate, pulled up behind me. Inside were four men. They were shouting out the window at me. Scared and startled, I thought how odd it was. I hadn't taken this to be a dangerous area. I sprinted off.

The car followed me, like you see in movies. And the men kept shouting at me. I was not taking it in. My receptive language is horrendous. I came to a massive main road which turned out to be the motorway. I thought, *Fuck – what now?*

Across the road I could see McDonald's and Costa Coffee. I thought, *If I can at least get to Costa, I'll phone the hospital and say these guys are chasing me.*

I waited for a gap in traffic, and sprinted to the central reservation, waited for another gap and sprinted to the other side. I thought, *Good. They can't get me now because they have to go way up the motorway to find a roundabout.*

I'm jogging down to McDonald's a few hundred yards away, and a huge police van pulls up. All these officers bundle out and smash me on the ground, handcuff me, and tie my legs up with restraints.

Having been relatively calm from home, at first I wasn't aware of what was going on. There was no overload before they assaulted me. But once I understood what was happening, I was incensed. I said, 'What the fuck are you doing? This is outrageous.' Then I must've gone into meltdown, because I remember little of what happened next.

I know that I was thrown into the back of the van. The lights brightly illuminated the cage I was in. My eyes screamed from their intensity. Handcuffs were cold on my skin and cutting in to my wrists. The leg straps were burning bands.

When I came around, I was back in the hospital in my room, tied up. I must've had an injection because I could feel my brain very fuzzy. I remember lying on the floor, crying, still handcuffed.

The police took the handcuffs off. I was totally sedated. I took my tennis ball and played with it against the wall in repetitive movements. This was predictable. It would come back to me. The doctor came in and put me on a Section 5(2). Bastards. I'd only been there a few hours.

After that I got this Section 2 for 28 days:

Nature and degree

The ASD presentation is associated with marked deficits in socio-emotional reciprocity (lack of empathy, intolerance of others, impaired theory of mind, and perspective taking); deficits in non-verbal communicative behaviours used in social interaction (difficulty interpreting other people's body language or emotions, low self-esteem) and deficits in flexible thinking and behaviour (rigid and obsessive thinking and behaviour, preference for routines and predictable activities and experiences and conversely tendency to emotional melt down due [sic] sensory overload).

Dangerousness

I am of the opinion that this is necessary in the interest of her safety and for the protection of other people. Miss Quinn genuinely wishes to have an assessment and appropriate treatment for her mental disorder [sic] however she is prevented from doing this due to the impact of her condition. Although she often states that she does not actually intend to kill herself or cause harm to others the intensity and sudden nature of these behaviours make them dangerous and difficult to manage under conditions of informal care. Miss [sic] finds the present treatment facilities. She has been provided with an annexe facility to reduce the impact of this [sic] however she still finds it intolerable.

My solicitor Jessica argued that I had been informal for eight months prior to my arrival at Falton Green and did well in York. They weren't interested in hearing that.

In York, they had taken me off all the drugs I was on. Here, they pumped me full of that shit again. Because I transferred from the acute unit, they used that medical chart. They wanted to give me haloperidol, which caused me to have tardive dyskinesia (involuntary, repetitive body movements e.g. grimacing, screwing up my face, and scrunching my nose), wreckedmy eyesight, and distorted my face.

My mum phoned the acute unit Clover and said, 'How dare you not tell them that she was contraindicated for haloperidol?' A formal complaint was made to the Trust, to which we received an 'I am sorry you feel that way' response from the CEO. Falton Green stopped giving it to me and it was contraindicated from then on.

It didn't take long to realise this autistic hospital was the worst place I had ever been. All the distressed people in there are majorly abused. Most have learning disabilities, so they don't even realise they're being abused.

I decided I wasn't going back on drugs. I had all my self-esteem. I said, 'I'm not taking your drugs, and I'm not staying in this room. Now give me the phone so I can speak to a solicitor.'

So, I phoned Jessica. She said, 'Oh, Alexis. I can't believe you're back on a section. You were doing so well. What happened?' I told her the whole story. I was in shock as I was telling her. Jessica agreed to take my case, even though I was 216 miles away. We liaised and prepared over the phone.

My life had gotten unbearable very quickly. I was put in long-term segregation because I had absconded a second time. I tried in vain to argue that they had broken the law. I said, 'This is completely unjust. I had every right to leave the hospital that day. I did nothing wrong. I was completely within the parameters of the law.'

I was in a lot of pain emotionally and physically from the ordeal of the run that went wrong. I lost hope. I just wanted to go back home. I hated being on 1:1 obs. I hated the smell inside. There was little stimulation. I wasn't allowed out, not even to the garden. I was in a glorified cage, treated worse than an animal. A day after I was brought back from the motorway by the police, I planned another escape.

I ran the same way but didn't get far. The police brought me back. Falton Green would lose funding for me if I left. They put me in long-term segregation, locked in that wing for six or seven days. I was on 2:1 obs. The two staff were arm's length even in the toilet and shower.

There was no table in the room so I had to eat off the floor. The food was cheap and disgusting, like from 1960s school dinners. It was always cold and completely unpalatable. I went back to eating cereal. But they ran out of milk and cereal all the time. They would only give me one pint of milk a day, and that had to include my tea milk. It was all about their budget, because it's a private hospital.

Usually, I was begging for water after about an hour of staff changing over. They changed every two hours, so sometimes I had to wait the entire two hours for food or water because they didn't want to open the door. When the staff would change, because I was on 2:1, four staff would come to open the door in case I tried to escape. I wasn't allowed outside. I was truly going insane.

I thought Clover was bad. This place was beyond bad. There was absolutely zero care. Nobody gave a shit. Working conditions were horrible for the staff, too. At least they were getting paid. One staff person left because of what they did.

After about two weeks of this, I had a tribunal. I waited patiently for this day. In the morning Dr Kutisha, whom I have since learnt is quite a prominent autism doctor, was my responsible clinician. In the two weeks I had been in Falton Green, I hadn't met him. I spent longer with the tribunal doctor than I had with Dr Kutisha. I was less than impressed.

Jessica came up from Morecombe Cove. Dr Kutisha presented his evidence first. He was sitting there saying I was a danger to myself and others. He didn't even know me.

Jessica asked, 'How long have you known this patient, Dr Kutisha?'

'Oh, I met her today.'

'So, you've known her as long as the panel has?'

'Yes. That's right.'

Then the nurse, Taisha, had to explain what happened. She didn't lie.

Ralph, the social worker, just talked shit about all the stuff I did way before York. He said, 'She definitely needs to be detained. She's dangerous, lacks insight into her condition, and she can't be controlled if she isn't on a section. We can't manage her.'

Jessica said, 'But she's been informal for seven or eight months.'

Ralph and Dr Kutisha said, 'Yeah, but she's dangerous.'

I was pleased that Nurse Taisha didn't lie or bend the truth. I obviously didn't agree that I was dangerous. Aside from that, she gave an honest account.

The panel discharged me. I decided I was going home for a break. Thomas picked me up.

I'd had no treatment, nothing, because I'd been locked in long-term segregation. I had psychology and occupational therapy for one hour a week only. I had no other therapy I was interested in, such as autism education and social skills training. Instead, I was tortured.

At this stage, I was reasonable. I'd been in York and at home. Overload wasn't my way of life yet. I was talking rationally, no dysfunction, no breakdown. I still had the stuff with Josh which I hadn't been able to think about.

The tribunal discharged me on the condition that I agreed to pursue treatment. I was at home for a week. As soon as I came back, I was put on observation.

There were two people, one sitting on either side of my bed, when I went to sleep. I wasn't allowed to put my hands in my pockets. They had to be visible at all times. I wasn't allowed to go to the toilet on my own, have a shower on my own, or go for a run on my own – even though I was informal. We negotiated that at weekends I could go home.

On Fridays, staff would drop me off at the train station in St Elphage. I would get the train into St Pancras in London – on my own. From there I would take the Tube to London Victoria and catch the train to Morecombe Cove, a three-hour journey

– on my own. I spent weekends at home with my daughter, and on Sundays I would make the same journey back to St Elphage and they would pick me up again.

As soon as I walked in through that door, I was put back on observation. Well, I'd had enough of this after a few weeks. Although I was used to people watching me take a shit, I didn't particularly enjoy it. I was fed up. I was humiliated.

I said to them, 'I want to leave.'

They said, 'You can't leave. You're not well enough.'

I didn't feel I had anything to stay in Falton Green for. The place was one of containment only. Most of the distressed people had learning disabilities. Sadly, I came to realise that if you had a learning disability and autism, you would likely be put in a place like this. I saw little hope from the staff for these people, and I didn't see many families supporting them either.

The therapy was rightly pitched at the majority, but that meant it was too basic for me. For example, in the community group we spent a whole lesson on when you go to town, what do you need to take? Well, a bag, a purse, a phone if you've got one. This was hard for me after such good therapy in York. I was hoping to learn how to manage overload in supermarkets, but we came nowhere near learning about something like that.

On my first lesson of cooking I was expected to cut all the vegetables, including onions and carrots, with a plastic knife. Seriously! I wasn't trusted to use a metal knife.

*

I was pleased for the mindfulness classes, something I had enjoyed in York. But after a few lessons from untrained staff not doing them properly, I offered to lead. I led quite a few groups. Then there was the DBT, one session a week. We read through the DBT skills worksheet. There was no application.

Again, I kept thinking I was weird. I didn't fit in anywhere. I didn't fit in mental health. I sure as hell didn't fit in there. I'd been given this diagnosis I didn't understand. I could see that I was autistic, and that others around me were too. It was incredible to observe the spectrum in such a way. In a hospital full of 40 people all with autism, you could see the same characteristics manifest themselves in very different ways. I felt as though I was with "my people" but I was so very different at the same time.

What was I staying for? I wondered. I was staying for an hour of psychology a week. That was it. I wanted to leave. 'No, you can't leave,' they would say. 'You're not well.'

I communicated this to my parents. In Falton Green, you're not allowed a personal phone so communication is very difficult. The staff cannot be without their phones. And on obs, staff is arms-length so there's no chance for open conversation. It's like being in the Big Brother house – and all this while I'm an informal patient. When I'd go out for walks, it would take a good 15 minutes to leave the building because they'd write down everything I was wearing and carry out a risk assessment.

I called my dad on one walk. He said he was coming to get me. I didn't think about his comment. I went to DBT. In the middle of the session, I was interrupted by an HCA and told to go outside. My dad was there. He said we were leaving, and we did.

*

At home, I was delighted to be back with Abi and to sleep in my own bed. I could even have the lights off and there weren't two people on either side of me. I slept well. I felt good. I reflected on Falton Green and realised that it was an awful place. I was nothing but a cash cow to them. The psychology from the facilities psychologist Alejandro was good, but that was it. There are 168 hours in a week and I couldn't stay there for 167 hours doing nothing just for the one hour of therapy I knew I desperately needed.

I talked with my GP and community psychiatric nurse and asked them to tell Falton Green to put a proper package together where I maybe went for a day a week. This couldn't be done. 'Why the hell not?' I was exasperated. 'It's cheaper,' I argued. Apparently, the funding was only for 24/7 care.

I felt so dejected. What on earth could I do? To make matters more irritating, if that was possible, I couldn't be put on the 12-month waiting list for psychology because I'd already had some and I wasn't "engaging with it".

This sparked a deeper interest in nooses. At home, I struggled with the lack of routine. It was an overwhelming change, the shift to doing things when I wanted. I didn't have to strategically plan my toilet trips around staff. I wasn't being watched when having a shower. I could go out for a run any time. I also found the memory of Josh's presence in the house difficult. He was conspicuous by his absence. I realised nothing had changed. I delved deeper into my special interest.

CHAPTER 40

European Vacation

I had been on section and missed so many holidays. I was really pleased when my parents took me with them to Europe for nine days. We managed to organise these trips in between admissions. It was difficult for my parents and I to understand my fluctuating capacity to function. However, what became clear was that my capability was mostly linked to sensory overload and the potential for meltdown – these concepts were not yet known to us and we didn't understand them. My parents regularly imposed restrictions on me in the hope of minimising the chance of meltdown, which didn't always go down well. We would fight about my curfews and grounding at my adult age. Fortunately, on this occasion, they were in agreement that I could travel.

We planned to watch my brother compete in the World Cup.

*

To get to the venue we drove across France and Switzerland. Our journey had been carefully mapped out and I knew what we would be doing every step of the way. I sat in the front and helped Dad navigate while my mum occupied Abi in the back. As always, Abi was immaculate in the car.

We visited castles, cathedrals, and museums on the way. The journey was beautiful as was the Swiss chocolate. Swiss chocolate-making standards have led the world since the early 1800s. It seemed important to try as much chocolate as I could. Abi didn't say no either.

In our spacious lodging in the Swiss Alps, I could watch cows grazing from the comfort of our sofa. I could also hear them. The cow bells, standard in this region, jingled and jangled from morning until night. I read that the purpose of a cow bell is to easily find the odd cow who might have wandered off for a nibble in that even greener pasture over yonder. I realised you couldn't possibly lose a cow with that thing tied around its neck.

Thomas raced and came fourth. He was disappointed, but resolute on winning in the World Championships later, which he did. I was pleased for him and so proud.

On the way home, we stopped at Parc Asterix. It's a theme park near Paris based on the comic book series *Asterix*. Much quieter than Disney, it incorporates themes from historic cultures such as the Gauls, Greeks, Romans, and Egyptians in the visual style of the stories. I was aware that these things would go over the head of a two-year-old. Even though the park was less stimulating than Disney, it was equally as fun. Watching Abi shy away from these larger-than-life characters wandering around, I saw how they could be scary to her. I thought if I saw someone so strange and 10 times the size of me, I might be wary too. I cuddled her into my top when I saw she wasn't getting used to them.

Abi loved the dolphin show. I did not. Yes, dolphins are impressive, intelligent, and athletic. But I wanted to see them free. I never thought this way before. I did now.

I didn't want to leave the place I was in. Not in the physical, mental, or the literal sense. Watching Thomas reminded me of my time as an elite performer and the thrill of competing on the world stage. Having the space away with Abi made me feel like a mother. I knew this feeling wouldn't last when I landed back in the UK.

CHAPTER 41

Seeing the Doctor

I'd been out of Falton Green a while and needed medication. I was addicted to the stuff. And under the mental health community team surveillance, I had to check in every three days. This time I went to the doctor. After a wait I headed upstairs, knocked on the door, and entered when the doctor called.

I sat down. She asked, 'How can I help you today, Alexis?' She smiled and was friendly. I explained I needed medication. She said she was not aware of my prescription and phoned the community team. When she got off the phone she said, 'I hear that you have left your placement.'

'That is correct,' I said.

'You still need help. You are ill, Alexis. Don't you know that?'

'I am not ill.'

'Alexis, do you understand your illness – what it means for you to be like this – to have autism and be vulnerable in the community?'

Wow, too many questions!

I chose one. 'Well, that is an interesting question, doctor. I'll answer in stages, and I will use a rhetorical question to start. What do you mean by illness? There isn't such a thing as mental illness. You are making it up.'

She interrupted me. 'Oh, Alexis, this is precisely why you need to be detained. You do not understand your illness.'

I didn't know what to say, so I started with an interesting fact I had read regarding the concept of illness. 'Did you know that there are more pathogens in your body than human cells? There is no indicator that pathogens cause mental illness. In fact, there is no scientific way to say whether I am ill or not.'

She looked at me. She said nothing. Her gaze was distracting me and felt awkward. I lowered my eyes to the floor.

'I am not suffering, you know,' I said defensively. 'I do not have an excessive domination of an emotional state. You can't argue that I do, so I am therefore not ill in that regard. To further support my argument, I have no functional interference, so I am not ill in that sense either. I am performing my functions as a homo sapien adequately.' She said nothing, so I continued, 'Do you feel that I am currently deviating in an unacceptable way from something I'm supposed to be doing? If so, I am unaware of it. Is this the case, doctor?'

'Now, Alexis, just listen to yourself. You are not making any sense. I think you are experiencing some psychosis,' she said. She pressed a button, which then turned orange, on her phone. 'You are jumping around all over the place not making any sense.'

I wasn't jumping anywhere. 'No, it is you who isn't making any sense. Please tell me why you think I am ill. Because I feel fine.'

'It's the way you are talking. You are not making regular conversation and you will not admit you are ill. That is a major problem. You need help. We are paying for you to get help at Falton Green and you have chosen to leave. You are clearly not well. That is not rational.'

'Well, now I understand what you consider to be illness. It took a while, but you got there in the end. Thank you for the clarification.' It was time for me to explain to her, so she could understand, so she could realise I wasn't ill, and that I had been treated badly. I mean, Falton Green had locked me in a room for days and treated me like an animal.

I continued my thread. 'You are misinformed. I was treated badly at Falton Green.' I thought it was best to get back to the point. Science is more effective than hearsay, so I returned to my argument which she surely would agree with. 'And you – you are using the functional interference model of human illness. Although this model can be helpful, you are failing to realise that you are placing moral judgement on the goal you have specified for me. It's not just you who does this, doctor. It's not your fault. Lots of people do it in a variety of ways. We allow systems, like in mental health in your case, to specify goals. Then you engage in a collaborative discussion like you just did on the phone. You discuss among yourselves what constitutes unacceptable deviations from the norm and voila ... you decide I am ill. Doctor, don't you realise you just did this with the mental health team?'

The doctor wasn't happy for some reason. 'You are being very accusatory, Alexis. It's unfair and it's aggressive. You need to accept your illness, show some insight and comply with the treatment you are being offered. You are not a doctor. You have no training. Do not tell me I am wrong. You have no right.'

How incredible! I continued fighting my case, but tried to talk more softly. I had been over-excited in my explanation and forgot certain etiquettes. 'I do know science, actually. My degree was partly science based. You are the one being clouded by moral judgement. It's simple. As soon as you start to define how I should behave, you define a goal as valid rather than just as a goal.' I laughed in triumph, and to try to make her laugh too. She didn't laugh.

I tried again. 'You are in an ethical realm, not a scientific realm, doctor.' I laughed and laughed. *Finally*, I thought, *I have explained myself.* I rarely got this far with a doctor because I was usually sent away. Doctors don't like to admit their concept of illness is incorrect because they think of themselves as scientists.

I laughed a bit more. The doctor told me she wouldn't be prescribing me drugs and would be recommending the community team visit my house. She pressed the phone again and the light turned off. I liked the rhythmical flashing.

She said, 'You have a mental illness that requires treatment. Do you at least understand that? If you can't even understand that, then I am going to recommend that the community team deal with you.'

I was annoyed. I felt I had explained myself well. Why didn't she understand what I was saying? I tried a different tack. 'Look, doctor. Not you, nor anybody else, can determine how things are the same and different. There are an infinite number of ways people can be, so they can't be categorised by objective similarity. There are no scientific categories of illness. Do you at least understand that?'

'Right, Alexis,' said the doctor. 'I am going to give you one last chance.' She pressed the button again. It flashed orange every second. 'Do you accept this drug for your illness? Do you accept you are ill and do you agree to go back to Falton Green?'

I was overwhelmed with the number of questions. I didn't know which one to answer first. Also, why didn't she agree with my line of thinking? How weird! I couldn't answer the questions, and she was getting off point. I decided to be more direct.

'Right, doctor. You don't understand what I'm saying. I thought you were smart but let me just help you. There are no precise categories for mental illness. So, no, I am not ill.'

The doctor picked up the phone again and called someone. Three people came into the room. This scared me. So, I continued, pretending that they weren't there. 'Think of triangles,' I said, trying to ignore my rising heart rate. I looked at the floor. 'This is important, pay attention: you can precisely define categories of a triangle because its inclusion and exclusion criteria are boundaries: it must have three sides, three angles, and the sum of its angles must add up to 180 degrees.'

I suddenly realised they were all talking over me. This felt rude, like children at school. I said, 'Excuse me, you need to listen.' I love scripts. They help so much. This one was a classic. When people talk over you, always remind them to listen.

'If the criteria for a triangle are not met, then it's not a triangle. This is called a "classical category".' I emphasised by using the gesture for quotations. 'When scientists work, they use "classical categories". But you, doctor, you do not do science. You are little more than a social engineer. Your whole book of so-called disorders is not classical categories. Do you get it now? You are a wannabe. You are trying to make me look ill when there is no such thing. So, to answer your question, *no, I am not ill.*'

'Alexis ... you know it all, don't you?' asked the doctor.

'No, not everything. But thank you,' I said, shocked by her admission. Something weird was happening because the other three laughed. 'It's not funny.' Another script from school. 'You see, psychiatrists by profession are trying to accomplish something that has a desirable end. They stupidly believe that what they are doing is science. They ask us patients to agree we have an illness and then agree to their treatment. Really their categories of illness are only *family resemblance categories.'*

'What are you going on about, woman?' said a small fat man. That was rude. He should have called me Alexis. I didn't correct his social etiquette, even though they regularly do that to me. I explained instead – it's far more productive. I had relaxed a bit about the three people in the room.

'It's simple. You know the way you have a "family resemblance" where, for example, there might be attributes that all your family members have but you don't have them all? That is called "family resemblance category". This is similar to the DSM.

It has lists of attributes for each category of illness. There will also be a rule about how many attributes you must have. The rule might be that you need five attributes out of ten to have the disorder. This means that person A could have the first five category descriptors, and person B might have the second lot of five. So, they share no features in common, yet they are members of the same category. That's a classic family resemblance category. The DSM is like this. There's a list of symptoms, and if you have enough of them you have the illness. So, you can see how silly it is to ask me to admit to being ill.'

Wow! I was vindicated. Until I stood up to leave. 'I would like my prescription now, please.'

'Alexis, I am afraid we have had to call the police. They will be here soon. Please don't worry.'

I ran out of the office the second she stopped talking and got the bus to Heysham. I bought rope and practised tying nooses. This calmed me. I saw a police car approach.

Now my head was in a spin. I couldn't speak. I tied the rope around my middle and hid it under my jumper. I paced and hit my hands together. Nothing would help me calm down. The police. The police. The sirens. The handcuffs. I was out the door. I ran and ran. Running past lamp posts, I started to count to six.

I didn't know what was happening. I was in handcuffs in the back of a police van with my knees and feet tied together. I was on the floor. I quickly calculated the dimensions of the van.

Then I was in the 136 suite ...

'Look, officer, this is very unjust. You are breaking the law. I am not on a section and I have committed no crime,' I said.

The officer said, 'You are detained under Section 136 of the Mental Health Act. You are a danger to yourself. We consider you are suffering from a mental disorder of a nature and degree that may warrant detention in hospital. You will be assessed soon.'

When I could speak again, which was after some time, I said, 'This whole thing started because I do not have a fucking mental health disorder. There is no such thing. They have diagnosed me because they want to treat me. But there is nothing to treat. The terrible problem is that every psychiatrist I meet insists on assuming the non-classical categories characterising psychopathology are classical. This is wrong and unscientific. I actually explained it to the doctor just a minute ago. Please ... they use the ICD or DSM, their bibles, based on pseudoscience, to enforce treatment that I don't need.'

'It doesn't matter what I see, Alexis. How many days have you been home? Less than a week. I don't know why they let you out. You are sick.'

'That is what they tell you. Do you want me to explain to you the system?'

'Sure, fill your boots,' said the police constable.

'What?' Then I realised he meant yes. So, I continued with what I was going to say. 'Right. So, in short, the psychiatrists gather a variety of people and assume homogeneity. This is as unethical as it is dangerous. You can't treat everyone the same. Ooh, sorry ... do you know what homogeneity means? In this context it means the diagnostic category is the same for everyone. But there is no homogeneity in a family resemblance category. The categorical structure for psychopathology is pragmatic and not scientific. I have no illness. They are mistaken.'

He just stared at me. He didn't answer. After a while, officer 6298 asked, 'Why did you run from us, Alexis, if you have nothing to hide? If you really are not ill?'

'Well, science would suggest that the amygdala, which arouses fear, accesses memories of things I don't understand or like. Such as mental health services and the police. It says to the rest of the brain something is wrong with this situation. It floods. Cortisol is released by the hypothalamus. This process puts me in a state of emergency preparation. If I'm in this state long enough, it makes me look as if I am mentally ill.' That's one theory I explained to him during the eight hours before the MH team arrived. Then they started their usual bombardment of questions I could never keep up with. I felt as though I was on fire. It became hard to concentrate.

'Do you want to harm yourself? Do you hear voices? Do you want to die?'

My response was the usual: 'No to all the above.' I waited for the next question. I'd been through this so many times. I knew what was coming.

'Do you think of suicide?'

'Yes, I absolutely do. I love the topic.'

'Do you want to harm yourself?'

'No, I just answered that.'

'Then why do you think of suicide?'

'Because the territory regarding the death of my brother is unknown. I'm in a state of unexplored chaos. My life since his death has been a cluttered mess. Because I cannot clean it up, I read about suicide. It's soothing. I think that's why. What do you think, doctors one and two, and social worker woman? Do you think that's correct?'

Doctor one replied, 'I'm not sure, I've just met you. Why don't you accept that you are ill, go back to Falton Green where you can get help, and agree to the treatment plan for your illness?'

'Oh, my gosh, do you people not share information? I ask this because I have explained countless times before … even in the last 24 hours I have explained to five different people. The answer, if you must have it again, is because I am not ill. However, if you want me to admit to something, then I will admit this very interaction causes the dysregulation you see. It is stressful. You are stressful. I feel threatened by you.'

'We are here to help you, Alexis. We can help you. Are you paranoid – worried we will hurt you?'

'No, I'm not delusional. Your help is locking me up for no reason. That isn't helpful. It makes me dysregulated. I want to go home.'

'Are you willing to work with services?'

'No. Not until services accept that human mental health is a matter of moral action more than anything else. No, I am not. All the pseudo-scientific crap in those places is a type of sin of omission designed as a shield to hide what the NHS is doing that is actually causing dysregulation. You are drugging me for no reason. You have no science to back up your assertions. Humans are not homogenous. I've explained this already.'

Doctor two added, 'If you do not agree to treatment, then I'm afraid I will have no choice but to section you.'

I do not know what happened next. I didn't store the bad memories of this time or other times. I don't think I even suppressed them. Experiences such as these are not nameable. It's so far outside the domain of what makes sense to me. It's so stressful I can't attach it to anything known in this world. I am not trying to deceive myself or hide things away. I know some patients who have not examined terrible events in their lives and this causes their pain. But I was not doing this. It's hard to explain. I try to grasp the nature of the category of things I don't understand and can't remember. It's a weird category that I will call potential. This potential is something I haven't been able to address because I don't know it and haven't had help to know. It's an unknown and unquantifiable stress. Woo-hoo – now that's how I conceptualise my "illness"!

*

Knowing that my life was over, I had melted down. I know this because I don't remember. Then I was in seclusion. I can't feel what happened or remember because it's too fast, and it hurts so much. All the lights get bright, everything is too loud, my body is on fire, and I scream. I know that in this moment I lost all hope and wanted to perish.

I must have been a real pain in the neck because I reacted so badly. But I argue with myself that I am not crazy. These events aren't normal. They mostly don't happen to people. If they happened to you, you might react like me. I am living in constant threat of trauma. This is all I have to try to make sense of it.

I sat there in seclusion pondering this idea. I needed to reconceptualise my recent past, not as a crazy person, but as a victim of terrible treatment, which included making me a mental patient. I mean, look at what had just happened.

In my hazy, drug-filled brain I reasoned something like this – the nurses and doctors were the ones deceiving themselves. They lived in these interpretive structures which provide a predetermined view of illness and reference point of normalcy. These structures they so loved are not complete. They do not reflect how the world really is.

It's ignorant, really. The problem is that what surrounds and contradicts their incomplete stories is a massive realm of possibility. The mental "doctor-scientists" are frightened that there are other ways to think about the world. There are ways to think of distress besides illness, faultiness, diagnosis, and treatment. It doesn't have to just be linear. That's what scares them. That's why they reject another view without listening. There are many ways people and the world could be if society acted in a different manner.

People are not a collection of objects with their own predetermined trajectories. People and real life are unconstructed possibility. Life can go in different directions, our futures malleable to an infinite degree.

My theory is this: if something happens to you so you behave in a way people consider wrong or sick or faulty, what you are experiencing may not be illness. It might be a set of influences. For things to improve, you must interact with that set of stimuli in society, not hospital, to learn from it about you and the world. This way you see how you construct yourself, and how you have constructed the world. You see how things might be different. With this understanding, you can make the changes you want.

According to my theory, you can't just put an interpretive framework on people and expect it to work; that's silly, because actual reality could be infinitely otherwise. That attempt is pathological. I am not.

*

I fell asleep.

Many hours later I was awakened by a doctor, a nurse, and two HCAs ushering me out of seclusion to my room in the 136 suite. *I will tell them about my musings later,* I thought. *Then they might understand.*

I was held under MHA Section 2, the 28-day assessment. I woke up a few hours later, and by caged transport, I was driven to Falton Green. I put up a real fight. There was no way I was getting in that cage easily. I cut my forehead as I fought.

I was on a 2:1 and again I wasn't allowed to go for walks. I hated my life so much. I phoned my solicitor, Jessica. We appealed to a tribunal and miraculously I won. But I had to stay at Falton Green and engage in treatment.

So, now I was an informal patient, I could go for walks in the country. I was on 1:1. Each day I would wait for the shift when the young HCAs came on and one of them could go with me. Most of the staff were in their early 20s, with little to no life experience.

I kindly explained to them, 'You're a baby. I used to teach children two years younger than you. Don't tell me what to do. You have no clue about life. You're not even qualified for this role. You don't have a degree or any training.' I was angry and fed up. I was done engaging in this so-called "treatment". Because the hospital was so poorly run, staff turnover was high. They recruited persons barely out of school to work for them, which led to the appalling care. Because they had no idea what they were doing.

Staff looked down on me and treated me like a sub-human. I started off with, 'Don't talk to me like that. Don't tell me to go to my room. Don't tell me it's time for bed. Don't tell me I need to change my clothes. Just don't speak to me.'

Invariably, they would chastise me. For example, I would be lying on my bed with my hands in my pockets. Staff, just because they could, would say, 'Get your hands out of your pockets.'

'Why?'

'Because your hands have to be visible at all times.' They'd say this to show they could control me. And they could control me. These were the people with power.

As always, a few staff were amazing. I played lots of Scrabble and taught others some backgammon. I organised my day around the staff rota. I'd decide who would take me into the garden, who would play Scrabble, who would play backgammon. Some I needed to avoid so I would read during their times.

After a few weeks, I had a good relationship with the kids. I told them, 'You should go to college. Do some social work.' A lot did. Two went to college, and one applied for a nursing programme.

I taught them yoga. Sharon, an HCA, stayed at arm's-length and we ran around the campus together. She was a lovely 40-year-old lady with two kids. She felt bad for me. She brought her running gear every day and we talked and talked. It was like having a friend and companion – she was good therapy.

I said, 'Sharon, it doesn't have to be like this. Don't work here, for a start. You shouldn't be spoken to like they talk to you.' Because of the running, she lost a lot of weight. That made me happy for her. But I wasn't there for them. Seeing as I was unlikely to be a world champion in Scrabble, I needed to get out.

I felt very depressed. The outside world didn't want me, thought I was a waste of space. And I was costing the NHS all this money. I was so high-functioning that I was a pain in Falton Green. They viewed me as a threat because I complained about the system and state of the place. I didn't want to go back to an acute unit, and I couldn't go somewhere like The Retreat. This Falton Green was apparently the best England had to offer, and it was dreadful. I couldn't stand one more night of the staff snoring and waking me up. I didn't want one more person to exercise any form of control over me. I didn't, as much as it pains me to admit it, want to see one more patient in distress. I'd had enough.

CHAPTER 42

The Plan

Mid-April 2015

When Sharon and I went for runs, I was timing to see how long it would take to get to a stream about a mile away. There was a lot of tree cover I hoped would block helicopter sighting. I spotted some rope in the garden. I calculated height and gradient on the river bank and found a strong tree branch. I visited it on my walks and runs for a few weeks.

I made an escape to time how long it would take me to get to the place I had in mind. One day when I was in the garden with staff, I hopped over the six-foot fence. I sprinted to the tree. It took 12 minutes. This was through fields with no access from the road. I made sure of that. I knew I had to get this right. It was my last chance really. Then I timed how long it would take to climb the tree. I didn't take the rope because obviously if I took it, I couldn't use it again. But it took too long to get up the tree.

I found a branch at the bottom where I could fix the rope. If I let it lie at a certain angle, I realised I could achieve asphyxiation. This spot was in the middle of a group of fields, but hidden. There was the motorway nearby, but that wasn't an issue because I'd be dead before they found me.

Nobody could get there in time. I calculated that if I could apply the noose within 16 minutes ...

When I was 100% sure of my plan I just stood there waiting for emergency services to arrive.

The police came. The police officer was very cruel. Officer 7885, I noticed. He said, 'You're a waste of time. You're a waste of space, you mental health people.'

'I'm so pleased that you're doing your job, officer.' I had learnt to use sarcasm.

'You are not my job. Catching burglars and murderers is my job.'

I said, 'Fuck off.' He drove me back.

The staff said, 'Don't do that again, Alexis. That wasn't good. What were you doing?'

I said, 'I was planning my suicide.'

'Oh, right, okay. So, how are you going to do that, then?'

'Well, I thought about using a rope, but it takes too long to climb up the tree. It will also be difficult to procure the length of rope I will need to break my neck.'

'How do you plan on doing it if you can't use the rope?'

'I'm just going to use my shoelace.'

'Right.'

The staff were fully aware of my plan. At the end of the week I went to see Dr Kutisha. He asked about the plan and I told him.

He said, 'Okay. Well, if you've made up your mind there isn't much I can do about it.'

I said, 'No, not really. I've decided that enough's enough.'

He says, 'Right, okay. That's fine then, Alexis. So, I'll see you next week.'

'No, you won't see me next week, doctor. I've just told you, and you're not listening again. You never listen. April 30th is my last day with you. I would love to tell you that it's been helpful here, but it hasn't.'

Still he says, 'Okay, I'll see you next week, Alexis.'

I was very confused by his reaction. Perhaps he meant that he'd see me when I was dead. I supposed that he might, so I say, 'Alright. Well, actually you might see me, but just not in this state.'

*

On 30th April I was in a care programme meeting. I said, 'Well, I'm not staying here any longer, with your authoritarian, restrictive, privacy-invasive practices, and on obs Monday to Friday, and then I suddenly and miraculously improve and can go home through Central London on weekends from Friday to Monday. I'm not doing it.'

'What are you going to do then?'

'I've told you. For goodness' sake, don't you people ever listen?'

'Okay, well .... '

After the meeting, I said goodbye to them all, and off I went. I carried out my plan. I sprinted off the campus. On the border of the field, Taisha was still with me. We had been running together for a few months and she was fit. She called to me, 'Alexis!'

I shouted, 'What, Taisha? What?'

She said, 'If you leave that field, you're going AWOL and your leave will be restricted. You won't be allowed out again. You know the consequences.'

Did she not listen either? Why would I need leave when I was going to be dead? I said, 'Bye,' and off I went, leaving her behind.

I jumped over the river, got to the branch, and applied the ligature. I was so very happy. I thought, *This is it.* I looked up, and there was a bright blue sky. It was such a tranquil environment, beautiful fields, right next to the river. I was leaning down the bank on the river. I had practised nooses a lot and knew how long it would take to go unconscious. It took two minutes for me.

Gradually, I felt the blood pooling in my head. Slowly, slowly I was going unconscious. The best way to describe the strangulation-type hanging is to compare it to when you're in a swimming pool underwater and you need to breathe. That pressure of needing air builds up. It was uncomfortable, but I was just so relieved. It was all going to be over. Finally, I could be at peace. The pain from the noose and pressure build-up was a reassurance.

I knew this was the only way. I was getting worse, and so depressed. The weekends at home – it was like I was being teased. *This is what you can have, but you can't.*

I knew the only reason I was in that place was money. I thought, *I've tried for two and a half years. I've been to so many services in this country. None can help me, so I'm clearly not supposed to be in this world.*

As I was going unconscious, I felt relieved that each part of the plan had worked. The lights went out.

*

The next thing I knew, I was lying on my back in the field, looking up at the sky which was no longer beautiful blue. I couldn't speak. I had those electrode things on my chest. I felt awful. My heart was beating out of my chest. All these people were standing over me, looking at me. There was a helicopter, propellers rotating.

They took me to the hospital and checked me over.

The police were there. Guess which policeman? Officer 7885. I said, 'Hello, 7885.'

He said, 'I'm sorry, Alexis. I'm so sorry.' I was sorry too. Sorry to be alive! Sorry to see that bastard policeman again.

After the physical health hospital, they took me to the 136 suite. I was completely empty. I had nothing to say, I was so upset. I knew I would get sectioned and spend years in hospital. How could I possibly have fucked up that badly?

There was one man who had been in Falton Green for nine years. Many people had been there over five. This was my fate and I felt it right to the core. And I had no way out now, because I'd be on too high obs.

I sat quietly, self-absorbed. My brain was full of emotions running around but no names for them. Nothing. Just nothing.

After a while, I spoke to the police. They were pleasant. Officer 7885 kept saying, 'I'm so sorry. I had no idea.' *No idea about what,* I thought? He explained that he just thought I was another time waster.

I said to him, 'The thing that you don't realise, 7885, is that I was a person before.' I told him my background. I explained that mental people, "crazy people" as he referred to them, are people. I told him the psychologist Eleanor Longden's advice. Instead of asking, 'What's wrong with her?' ask, 'What happened to her?' Do you see the dynamic shift?

He said, 'I didn't know, Alexis. We come across so many people in these 136s – attention seekers.'

I said, 'Yeah, but these so-called attention seekers all have a story. They don't just land in here for no reason. Everybody has a story, and mine isn't any more tragic just because I was a PE teacher, a professional person, or have been to university. How far I've fallen doesn't make me any more of a tragic case.'

I could see that my words made an impact on him.

I told him, 'The worst thing is my life is about to get a whole lot worse now. It's worse because of psychiatry.'

'What can I do?'

'The thing you can do is next time you get called to a 136, don't treat the person like shit. There's a reason people land here.'

He said, 'Okay, but how can I make it better right now? I'll tell you what. We're going to get a McDonald's.' I had told him how bad the food was at Falton Green. So, he phoned up on his police radio, and requested a McDonald's order to the 136 suite.

In about half an hour, the McDonald's came. And the MHA officers arrived. There were two doctors and a social worker. They were busy ignoring me and the police and talking with each other.

I said, 'I can't even fucking enjoy my McDonald's, 7885.'

He says, 'Yeah, you can. Listen, you'll get sectioned anyway. Just have fun in there. Every time they ask you if you're suicidal, slurp your drink. Every time they ask if you have thoughts of harming yourself or other people, chomp your burger. And I'm going to do it as well.' That made me smile. For once I was grateful for the police.

*

We were sitting in the 136 suite. The doctors entered, serious. 'Alexis, we've been called here today because you've had to be resuscitated due to a suicide attempt. Why did you do that? Do you think you will do it again? Do you hear voices?'

Too many questions, but for once it didn't matter.

I went, slurrrp, slurrrp. They were looking at me. I said, 'Definitely.'

They said, 'So, if we let you go today ...'

'You're not going to let me go.'

They said, 'Yes, but if we let you go, are you going to try to commit suicide?'

I said, 'Absolutely.' Chomp, chomp, chomp. And 7885 was doing it as well.

For once in these assessments, I was relaxed. I wasn't overwhelmed. I was put at ease not by the mental health team or the psychiatrists, but by 7885. I had an hour of relief with those guys. I was mindful like I had been taught in York, just staying in the moment. And I enjoyed every bite of that burger.

I was sectioned. But it was a Section 3, a six-month treatment section. I needed treatment apparently. I agreed. I did need help. Good, well-structured, caring treatment, not torture. I had to be taken back to Falton Green. The police asked, 'Do you want us to take you, Alexis? We're due off shift.' They had been with me about eight hours, through their whole shift.

'No, I'm not going in there willingly.'

'Look, we'll just take you. It's no trouble. We'll take you now, and you can have a little bit more time.'

'No, it's fine.'

They said, 'Okay, we'll come and see you next Friday.'

So, they took me back to Falton Green in a caged ambulance. I didn't resist. I went in willingly. I was on serious obs and wasn't allowed outside, even to the garden. The 30th April was a Thursday. I had the whole weekend without being allowed out of my room.

I was so embarrassed. I found it hard to talk to staff at all. I didn't know what to say to them and they didn't know what to say to me. I had never really failed before in my life. This failure was of epic proportion. I was so sure, telling the doctor, 'You won't see me next week.' Afterwards, I held my head in shame.

Falton Green issued my care coordinator from my home county with 28 days' notice to leave. Here are the clinical notes from the call:

01/05/2015 12:27:00 Knight, Elaine

CC CMHT – Call received from Olumide, staff nurse at Falton Green.

Alexis was found by police in a helicopter with a ligature around her neck, hanging from a bridge. She required resuscitation by police and was transferred to the general hospital. She has since returned to Falton Green and is now under Section 3 of the Mental Health Act.

Alexis is currently pacing around the unit and is asking staff if she can leave to go out for a run. This clearly is not deemed safe for her to do.

Herbert Ledstone, the manager of the therapeutic campus, and I wrote to them and asked for me to stay in Falton Green, because the consequences were high. But they said no. I think it was just a ploy to get in writing positive attributes.

I wanted them to let me go. Of course, they didn't let me go. I knew that within those 28 days an ambulance would come for me. They wouldn't tell me if they were going to do it in the night. I had difficulty sleeping.

And for the first couple of weeks, they wouldn't tell me where I was going. It was a mind game. They knew. Dr Kutisha had put in an application for a forensic assessment. The letters and referrals had been sent to the Trust. They were angling for a low or medium secure. Dr Kutisha told me to expect medium secure. He said I wouldn't be going out at all, and the fence would be 5.2 metres high. 'You won't be jumping over that fence, Alexis,' he said and he smiled as he spoke. Such a nasty guy. I wished that I was dead.

I had to sleep with the light on. The two staff always went to sleep sitting beside me. I'd have my ear defenders on, and they would be snoring right next to me. They didn't care. They closed their eyes, slept for 10 minutes, then got up and carried on.

One night, an HCA named Benevolence just kept snoring. I was so furious that I clapped my hands as loud as I could right beside her ears. She couldn't complain about it because she'd been sleeping.

If I could have tied a noose, I would have. I made nooses from anything, from my trousers. It's a real talent. Seriously, I'm amazing. If it wasn't viewed as so weird, if from the moment Josh died they had just accepted my interest in death, didn't make it into a hugely strange thing like I was an unemotional monster, it would have gone a long way towards averting this. You have to realise when you marginalise somebody's interest, especially on the back of a massive bereavement, that's going to have an impact.

Now I don't talk about this interest at all to anybody. I learnt to shut up. But when I started this journey, I thought the psychiatrists were trying to help so I told them everything. It's a strength to be honest, not to have to think what someone else is thinking and be able to talk freely. It's also a massive weakness, because people can exploit that. I learnt in these four years to be more careful.

On the next Monday, I hadn't been outside for more than a week. I said to them, 'If you don't let me into the garden, I'm going to speak to my solicitor and tell her you are breaching my human rights. I have the right to fresh air. Even prisoners get an hour a day. If you can't manage my risk in a humane way, then you need to move me now.'

They allowed me into the garden. But I had to be in level-one holds, with two staff holding my elbows and my wrists and pressing them right to my body. I had to walk in restraint in the small garden.

I needed to move. The restraint hurt me badly because of the touch, and they knew that. Sharon, the first couple of times she had to do it, was tearful. We walked around for the 10 minutes I was allowed, with Sharon constantly apologising. She was a star. Sharon ran with me around the garden in the holds after a while. She would get another kid who liked to move and we would run together. What a wonderful woman. Sharon kept me going. She kept me hopeful and alive in spirit.

'I'm sorry about this, Alexis. Really I am.'

I pleaded. I begged. 'I'm not going to escape. Just let me go. I promise you I won't escape. Just get off me.'

They said, 'We can't. You either cooperate with the restraint or we can't be out here.' So, it was like that for four weeks.

The police did visit me on the first Friday, seven days after I was sectioned. I was tearful when I saw them. I had misjudged 7885, and he had misjudged me. We sat in the garden. I had staff attached to my arms while 7885 and the female officer sat on the other side of the bench. They were in shock. They asked, 'Why do you have to hold her like that? You know it hurts her, right? We're here, let her go while we talk. Give her some space for a private conversation.' Staff didn't.

The final month in Falton Green was just horrendous. That place was disgusting and dirty. I can't even describe it. They never cleaned up Fiona's vomit. I remember once I went to the toilet upstairs. I lifted the toilet lid and my hand was covered in sick. I went to get in the bath, and it was covered in sick and toothpaste. So, I went downstairs, and they handed me a bucket and told me to clean it myself. And those women are still in there. There's no more wrong with them than there is with me. They are autistic and think differently. That is all, in my opinion.

I had no incidents for the 28 days I waited to leave. They threatened me by saying they would send me to medium secure. I was scared. So were my parents. That is why my parents wrote the letters asking for me to stay. In the end, I went to intensive care.

I was transferred back to Ivy Suite. An ambulance arrived on 28th May, 2015. Two HCAs went with me to PICU. They didn't touch me and let me walk inside by myself. When we arrived at PICU, there was nobody to meet us outside because they were busy. Normally, you're supposed to be kept in the ambulance, in the cage, until someone comes out. The HCAs let me out and I showed the "kids" around the hospital. This confirmed what a mockery it was.

I have never been so happy to see Ivy Suite. Nurse Achala met me in reception. She hugged me for a long time. I really needed that, and the pressure felt nice. She said, 'We're happy to have you back, Lexi.'

CHAPTER 43

Dear Ivy Suite

28th May 2015

Getting back to PICU was wonderful. I never thought I'd say that. I was so happy to see Achala. It was nice for me that she was shocked at how different I was. It's remarkable what had happened to me since I was last in Ivy. When she saw me before, I was a wreck, constantly in overload, a total nightmare to manage because of all the meltdowns. And the last time she saw me, nobody understood why an apparently capable person kept flipping out.

Before I arrived, all of my information had been sent from Falton Green. PICU is well staffed so the whole team read everything. This is not common. In acute units, where probably a third of the ward is coming and going every few days, staff don't bother reading the information because they haven't got time and the new person will leave soon anyway. In PICU, the success of their care depends on staff knowing everything and working with the person, usually for at least six weeks.

When I turned up again, they had my sensory report, my speech and language and my autism reports. I walked in calmly, not sedated or in overload. I was feeling lighter than usual because I was so relieved to get out of Falton Green. I sat down with a new nurse named Choki.

I spoke to Choki and quickly learnt that he was Japanese and from Tokyo.

'I used to live in Sumida near Tokyo Tower,' I told him.

'Oh, I lived in Shinso just over the river from there!'

'That's amazing!' It felt good that we had something in common.

Choki and I began work on my care plan. It was the first time since York, eight months before, that I sat with somebody whose intent was to help me put a detailed plan in place. This team spent two or three days writing the report, and I was included. They set goals and ways for me to manage. We signed every part of the care plan. I had one for sensory, one for speech and language, one for meltdown, one for food and drinks.

This made me feel brighter. Staff understood me. It was a good plan because it was achievable, one that worked and made my life tolerable. I think it was the first time intensive care assisted me in an informed way. Before it had always been a shot in the dark. Now armed with a diagnosis and understanding, the care plan could target specific needs.

The annoying thing was that I'd come on a 2:1. But at least Achala said, 'I'm really sorry, Lexi, but we're going to have to put you on a 1:1 because your risk level is so high.'

'I'm not really risky, Achala. It's fine.' That wasn't strictly true. I felt fine but was still very sad.

She said, 'No, we have to. If you don't have any incidents for 72 hours, Dr Saty will take it off.'

My relationship with the staff was amazing. I felt immediately at ease because they were genuine and honest. Everything was done compassionately there, even restraint. When they had to restrain, they usually did it in a seclusion room. If they injected, they did it in the bedroom. They didn't make you suffer in public.

That night, I asked the 1:1 if I could have hot chocolate. It's my routine to have a hot chocolate before I go to sleep. That was my routine for six months in Falton Green, and eight months before in York. Everybody in Falton Green had a hot chocolate before they went to bed.

He said, 'No, I'm sorry. You can't have hot drinks at night.'

I said, 'But look, I really need a hot drink, so could you just get one? It's not an issue. It will take two minutes. Please.'

'No, sorry, it's the rules.'

'Well, it's not the rules because I was here for months before. I know it's not the rules, and I know I'm allowed a hot drink before I go to bed.' This was an agency nurse, someone who rarely worked in Ivy – someone who couldn't be bothered.

'No.'

'For fuck's sake! Can I have some water then?'

'No.'

I went to sleep but woke up quickly because my mouth was dry. I genuinely needed a drink. I'd been running all day during the hourly courtyards. I was so happy to run 17 paces up and down that pesky courtyard. Thank you so much, NHS. You're amazing. These simple things matter when you have nothing. Like looking at the sky and breathing in fresh air that doesn't smell of Fiona's sick.

I needed to drink so badly. 'You've got to get me a drink. Let's go.' Between midnight and six o'clock in the morning you weren't allowed out of your room. I said, 'Just call someone to get a drink. If you don't want to move, that's fine, I'll stay here. I'm not asking you so I can get out of my room. I am happy to stay in my room. I just want to drink.'

'No.'

'Give me some fucking water now. You need to give me a drink, or I'm going to see the nurse,' I said. 'Alright. I'm going to see the nurse.' He blocked the door.

'Get out of the way. You can't keep me in here. This is like imprisonment. It's not a seclusion room. Get out of the way.' So, he moved a bit and I went out the door.

I tried once more, 'Mate, just give me a cup of water.'

'No.'

He pressed the alarm. I don't know what happened next. I do know I spent the whole night, from one o'clock in the morning until six o'clock in the morning, in seclusion. I got so drugged for that. I hadn't had an incident for 28 days, since I'd hung myself, and I had no drugs. I had a really good sleep in seclusion.

When I came out in the morning, I said, 'Right, give me a pen and paper.' I wrote a complaint.

Mishan was the ward manager. He came to see me. 'You should have been given a drink. You are allowed a hot drink. I apologise. It won't happen again.'

'Do you know how bad it was in seclusion for five hours with no water and totally drugged? It's unacceptable.'

Mishan was genuine. He treated me with respect and didn't try to cover it up. He didn't blame me. He was matter of fact, and he apologised. What more could I say? I thanked him for that. I didn't take it further. They meant no harm.

Shyam and other staff knew if I was melting down it was out of my control. This was a big step forward. I was given the time and space to learn what was difficult and to find solutions.

The staff helped me by stepping up the sedation drugs. It worked. Being sedated isn't a great way to live, but it meant I could manage the environment better. One uncomfortable thing about having so many injections is that you get a big lump at the injection site where the muscle swells. It's painful. They'd say, 'Alright, go to your room. Let's do an injection.' If I had complained, I knew that a) they would've done it anyway, b) I would never have gotten out of there, and c) they were doing it because they cared, not because they wanted to have an easier life. It wasn't like that with this Ivy Suite staff.

This was the best five weeks I ever had in Ivy Suite. But it wasn't all roses. Even today, I have a circle of pinholes on both bum cheeks from the injection points.

But they shouldn't have had to sedate me. They had to show that my risk had decreased. Because just five weeks before I had hung myself, they had to show they had met all their targets for reducing risk. I understood that.

Even though I was still held against my will, I was freer than I had been in a long time. I had time, space, and support to explore my autism. I used the sensory room for the first time. I was allowed in there a lot because it was in my care plan. Falton Green is for autism and they didn't even have a sensory room! I would sit in Ivy, staring at the bubble tube, watching it change in its predictable colours, and I'd feel at peace ... even if it was short-lived.

There was a funny woman in Ivy on this admission named Eileen. She was Irish, about 55, with long, silver hair. Eileen was a jovial, gregarious lady. She was fat, with massive breasts and skinny legs. She thought she was married to Prince Charles. She appeared normal otherwise. When I first met her, I couldn't identify her distress. I wondered why she was in intensive care. She was there before me and remained for months after.

One day, I was talking with Eileen about families. Suddenly she switched from her Irish accent into a posh English accent. It was amazing. 'Prince Charles and I have 13 children.' She was completely convinced.

I asked her, 'Where do you live?'

'Oh, Alexis, don't you know? We live in Kensington, dahling.' She did this all the time. And she might say, '... and that bitch, Camilla.' Her reality was a happy one and so detailed. She might say stuff like, 'I'm awfully proud of young William.'

She would flit in and out of talking about her "husband" and "children". I felt sad because I thought, *Who are they to say her reality is wrong.* She just thought she was married to Prince

Charles. Because her reality is different, why must we lock her up and drug her?

This was the first time I questioned compulsory detention. I hadn't thought about it so strongly before. Obviously I hated it, but I had been brainwashed into thinking I was ill and encouraged to agree it was necessary. I didn't feel this way about Eileen. She was happy in her reality and what was so wrong about that?

Everyone thought I was crazy because I kicked off the most. But I learnt to manage the effect of the environment much better in Ivy. Because the staff ratio was so high, someone would say, 'Okay, Lexi, it's getting noisy. Shall we go over to the TAU to play table tennis?'

They would notice minor behaviours like subtle stims or my accent changing. When my brain is too full, my words get clipped. Staff said, 'Lexi, we're noticing this. Can you not recognise it?' Only then, I would notice. That's when they would suggest we play Scrabble or backgammon. I got good at Connect 4, because I can see patterns. It's a short game, less than 10 minutes. When my concentration was bad, I would coach the staff. So, when I became non-verbal, they would get the game out. It's reassuring because it's predictable, like chess. I never lost a game because I could work out the patterns.

If it hadn't been for Shyam and Achala, I would've stayed in a negative emotional state. In Falton Green, I was just waiting to kill myself. Even when I arrived in Ivy Suite, although the feeling wasn't as strong, I was still waiting. After probably a week in Ivy, I didn't feel like I needed to die. I think it was their humanity and compassion.

Soon, I learnt that the Trust was trying to find me another placement. I had forgotten that when I left Falton Green, the referral had already gone in for a forensic assessment. However, Dr Saty, although sympathetic to medium secure, wanted to see how things played out. He said he would give me a chance to explore acute. If I didn't improve, it would be medium secure.

Meanwhile, a private locked unit in London had been asked to assess me. This unit was in the NHS so it would be a faster and cheaper place for them to send me. It would free up much-needed bed space, and they would be seen to be providing treatment.

Shyam told me that later that week I would be assessed. He came with three people from the locked unit. They interviewed me. Their service was totally inappropriate. I said, 'No, I'm not going to engage in your service.'

'Well, you can't come if you're not going to engage.'

'I'm absolutely not going to engage. I've done so much mindfulness in York that I could teach you. And I could teach you DBT as well. I know Marsha Linehan. I can tell you what's written halfway down on page 37 of the *DBT Skills Training Manual of* ISBN number 9781462516995. I will go with you, but I refuse to engage.' I stood up for myself.

They said, 'You're definitely not suitable.'

Shyam, I'm sure, was trying to contain a laugh. He knew I wanted to go back to the community. At the end, he whispered, 'Nice one, Lexi. You talked yourself out of that.'

Commissioners do this. They reallocate money to wherever can take you the quickest to get you out of acute services.

Dr Saty gave me leave to see Abi for two hours a week. This was like gold. No patient got that much time. The most Section 17 you can have is 30 minutes. I felt so lucky. My special interest changed to *Game of Thrones,* and Shyam let me watch it in the TV room on my own. I'd watch it over and over. I also read the books and memorised house lineages. He was a fan too, and we discussed it.

The only worrying thing that happened in Ivy Suite on that stay was that they gave me too many sedative jabs in 24 hours. My heart rate went down to 34 beats a minute. I managed to say to Shyam, 'I'm feeling really funny.' Then I fainted. I was semi-conscious when they wheeled me out on the stretcher.

I was rushed to hospital in an ambulance. After they gave me adrenaline to raise my heartbeat, I woke up there. I was scared. I had to keep my legs up in the air for ages. The recommendation from the physical doctor in the hospital was, don't give her so many drugs. I nearly died.

It wasn't long before I had a CPA, care plan meeting with Dr Saty. He successfully argued that I should return to acute, and then go back to the community. I think he noticed a big change in me and saw I was motivated to get back to real life. I didn't identify as "ill" any more. I had avoided forensic services once again.

CHAPTER 44

Henry is Too Tired to Do His Job

1st July 2015

The night before I left, Shyam said, 'Lexi, I have amazing news.'

'What? What?'

'I've got you a bed in Heysham.'

'That is amazing. What ward is it?'

'Blackthorn hospital, Oaken Ward. The ward that is joint to Primrose.'

'I know it. I've been on it before. Shyam, thank you so much.'

The next day Achala was on shift. I said to her, 'This is truly the last time I'll see you.'

'Really? You say that every time, Lex. But this time I know it's going to be the last time.' She gave me a hug, and off I went in a taxi.

I arrived on the ward, and it hadn't changed. Beneath the shine of the still new surrounds, garden and ward furniture, was the substandard treatment. The doctors were on holiday, of course. It felt as though these psychiatrists were always on holiday.

A junior doctor admitted me. I immediately asked for my Section 17 leave. I was only a few miles from my daughter and was eager to see her. I told him, 'Please, you need to get a consultant in here to do the Section 17.'

He started, 'Oh, I don't think …' I knew what he was going to say. It's not possible.

I said, 'No, it is possible. Just get a psychiatrist from the next ward. It's a two-minute walk across the courtyard. I need to see my daughter. I need to go outside and run. I've been in intensive care for five weeks, and before that Falton Green and have not been properly outside.'

In the end, the junior doctor phoned Primrose and asked the consultant to walk the two minutes over to Oaken to give me leave. That was kind.

The consultant turned out to be the one and only Dr Dempsey. I was actually surprised she came. She wrote me up for 45 minutes. I was grateful.

I couldn't help but notice how procedural Dr Dempsey was. How uncaring and matter of fact. She had been asked to write up leave, and that was clearly all she was going to do. She didn't ask how I was, she didn't ask what I had been doing the past two years. She didn't ask how York had been. She asked nothing aside from what she needed to ensure I wouldn't kill myself. I was reminded that I was nothing. Merely a different species with a diagnosis, who wasn't worthy of decent human interaction.

I said, 'Dr Dempsey, good to see you.' No response. 'And just so you know, I haven't been in forensic. And I don't have a personality disorder. I have autism.' I wanted to make these points to demonstrate to her I wasn't what she thought I was. I was not a ticking time bomb.

Her reply, 'Okay, so 45 minutes then?'

'That will be fine, thanks.' What was the point of expressing my dissatisfaction any further? I was keen to get outside and enjoy my "freedom". I took the copy of the Section 17 and went to find an HCA to take me out.

I went out with an HCA called Henry. My 45 minutes included getting to walk to the shop off the hospital grounds. Henry was about 30 and fairly fit, so we got a decent walking pace on.

We were just about to leave the grounds and he said, 'We're not going off hospital grounds.'

'Well, we are.' I referred him to my leave form from Dr Dempsey that stated I can go off hospital property.

'No, you don't have leave for off the hospital.'

'Henry, I know I've got leave. I'm not one of the people who doesn't know what day of the week it is. I've just been given leave. That's why we're going out.'

'Well, I don't want to walk to the shop. I'm really tired.' Henry was an agency staff person, which meant he didn't always work for the hospital. Agency staff, to make more money, do many shifts. For example, they might do a night shift in one hospital and then work the day shift in another. This isn't conducive to quality care.

I told him straight, 'We are walking to the shop, Henry, because I haven't been outside for three months. For this next 40 minutes we're going for a walk, okay?'

Then he grabbed me on the wrist. I froze. I said, 'Get off.'

He shouted to another HCA, Ruby, who was seeing somebody off in a car. We were not yet off the grounds. I knew Ruby well, and I said, 'Ruby, tell him to get off me. He's assaulting me.'

She came over, and of course she helped him. Now I had two people on me. Just as this happened, an ambulance drove past. The ambulance stopped and all the crew bundled me. Now I was in overload. Henry pressed his alarm. Many people came running from inside.

They tied me to a stretcher, including my head. I was going nuts. I was strapped immobile. I couldn't move anything; my heart was beating out of my chest and every part of my body was on fire.

Henry said, 'Shall we wheel her up?'

The ambulance crew said, 'No, let's put her in the back of the ambulance.' So, they wheeled me into the ambulance, and drove me up to the ward. I remember thinking, *I can't believe this is happening.*

I couldn't move my head, but I could hear the ward doors open and see bright lights shining powerfully overhead. I was wheeled through the airlock. I felt the intense entrapment as the airlock doors thudded closed after the stretcher. Everyone was watching. There was special interest because of the ambulance crew escort. Patients crowded the stretcher. I wanted to shout out something, but I managed only a scream.

They took me into the calming room. I pressed my body against the straps, but I was strapped down tight. My heart was like a frog inside jumping frantically to escape.

The deputy ward manager, named Jade, came in. She said, 'Let's just leave her on it because it's easier than restraining her.'

The ambulance crew said, 'Well, we need to go, really. We were just passing.'

So, they took me off the stretcher, moving me onto a heavy couch covered in plastic leather. Four staff then leant up against me, pressing me into the back rest of the sofa using their backs and torsos as leverage. I was fully restrained again, including my head. And I had been injected. Gradually, I calmed down. I was exhausted and meandered to my room and slept and slept. I was without spoons.

I went to see Jade some hours after. I said, 'I want to phone the police and make a complaint about Henry because he assaulted me. He caused that whole incident because of his laziness.'

'Henry's told me what happened, Alexis. He said you were trying to run in the road and throw yourself in front of cars.'

'If I had wanted to run, there's no way that man would've caught me. You know that.'

'Well, the other thing you have to bear in mind is that if you make a complaint to the police about Henry, then no one's going to want to take you out on Section 17 leave.'

I said, 'Fine. But listen. I know what happened, he knows what happened, and I'm sure you know what happened, because you know logically that if I wanted to run in front of a car, I could. So, you can threaten me, but you know the truth. I hope what you have done haunts you. You people make me question humanity.'

So, I didn't make a complaint. I value my walks and I needed the pseudo-freedom they offered. I remember Shyam and Achala saying, 'The future is in your hands'. In this instance, it was. I chose to put up and shut up.

I felt the true difficulties of being autistic on a mental health ward. I wasn't sick. And actually, looking at most people there, they weren't sick either. What good is the system doing?

CHAPTER 45

Desensitisation

I saw my first restraint within 24 hours of being on an acute ward. All the alarms went off. The staff went running. I heard a distressed person screaming and the staff shouting. I saw everything because they wrestled the person to the ground in the social area. I was shocked and very tearful. It's rare that things affect me that way.

Restraints are a "normal" part of life in a psychiatric hospital. The restraints you didn't see were the planned ones, like when I got Accuphase. Staff did those in the bedrooms. Sometimes you could hear through the walls the screaming and resisting of the distressed person.

Restraint isn't always used to manage violent incidents. It's most often to enforce detention and treatment. In an inpatient unit, people are continually restricted; doors are locked, clothes can be removed, jewellery taken away. This understandably produces a reaction. Then staff expect these people to take medications that make them feel a whole lot worse. It's like mind prison. You have no choice but to take the drugs or risk them being administered by force. This draconian practice has full backing of the law.

When I was last in the acute unit, I remember being shocked at how I'd changed. One day the alarms went off for a friend,

Peter, from Slovakia. His diagnosis was schizophrenia. Peter was small and muscly, but because of the antipsychotics they gave him, he had a massive belly. Peter was in constant motion from his decade of care and side effects. He had tardive dyskinesia and was always rocking-rocking-rocking – backwards and forward, backwards and forwards. When he was standing, he shuffled his feet.

I'd known Peter for a while. He was a good-looking man with blue eyes and high cheekbones. This day I was sitting in the canteen and he lined up to get his food. He was a big eater because of the olanzapine. Every day Peter would eat a full plate of mashed potato at dinner. The server behind the desk threw the plate at him. Peter swore a lot because his English vocabulary was limited. He said, 'What the fuck are you doing, ma'am?'

Instead of the HCA de-escalating it, she said, 'Don't speak to me like that. Don't be aggressive. Don't you swear at me.' Then she stared him right in the eye and pushed the alarm. It blasted **doot-doot-doot-doot**. So I thought, *Oh man, here we go.*

Staff came running. Peter was aggressive when people went for him. When you have four to six people running at you, it's flight or fight. Peter immediately was punching and kicking out at the staff. He landed a punch on the ward manager, Akachi. I sat on the chair and put my feet up on the table. I just watched, and rightly or wrongly I thought, *That's hilarious.* I couldn't believe Peter had taken on four staff and was trying to beat up the ward manager. Many of the other distressed people watched as well and were probably thinking the same. It was only the newbies who were still sensitive.

In the end five people restrained him on the floor for ages, putting their bodies over his limbs – his head, both arms, both legs. Then he went into what looked like an epileptic fit. Still, beside the other ward occupants, I sat there with my feet up, watching the entertainment.

When it was all done, I said, 'Ah, Pete.' I gave him a hug and said, 'That's cool, mate. She was a bitch, wasn't she?' We just sat there. He had been in for years and years.

He said, 'Yeah, what a bitch. At least I punched Akachi.'

I said, 'Yeah, that was cool.'

That's how you get through it. It happens to staff as well. You see them start off all compassionate and there for the right reasons. I saw it so many times with the young student nurses who came in. I used to call them Pearl, because they were so sparkly, shiny, and new. Within a few months they changed. Otherwise it would get them down, wouldn't it? They become hardened.

CHAPTER 46

What to Do with Me?

I was still on section. They didn't want to remove the section for some reason. Staff actually said, 'We just don't know what to do with you.' The four months I was there I got more and more distressed. That is not how "treatment" is supposed to work.

When I left Ivy Suite, my special suicide interest had been well under control. I was *Game of Thrones* obsessed. It was mainstream and I didn't feel so bizarre.

As I stayed in acute, the suicidality obsession became stronger. I delved into it and studied things I didn't know. I felt again like I didn't belong on this earth. I felt like I was an alien, or some other crappy cliché. I looked for clues about Josh as I studied.

My mood didn't go unnoticed. I couldn't even take a poop without somebody noting it, so the fact I was feeling low was recorded. The doctor started me on sertraline, an SSRI, because they thought I was depressed. I said, 'You've started me on sertraline three years after my brother died. Did you not think I was depressed three years ago? Is it not normal for me to feel depressed under my circumstances? If I was happy, wouldn't that be more worrying? Surely, I should feel the way I do.' The dose was increased.

Soon I developed asthma. It turned out to be caused by the sertraline. When I came off sertraline much later, the asthma completely disappeared. When I told them I had never had asthma, that something was causing it, they didn't care.

Looking back, I don't think the sertraline made me feel any better, because I wasn't pathologically depressed. I was just autistic and responding appropriately to an awful situation.

I looked up the chemical imbalance theory, which is the reason they prescribe SSRIs. I also made it my business to research these drugs. There is zero evidence to support that there are chemical imbalances in the brain. It's a theory drug companies use to sell their products. For all the money the drug companies spend on research, they would know by now if there was a chemical imbalance. This would help them even more to sell their products. It's just a load of crap. I didn't want a lot of their bloody drug, but they made me have them.

I had been on a Section 3 for three months and they wouldn't remove it. I would stay detained unless I won my tribunal. But all my doctors puzzled, where should she be detained? And the next question, who wants Alexis?

The lovely Dr Felicity Hart reappeared and decided they should send me to rehab.

'I'm not going. I don't need rehab. What do you do in rehab, anyway?'

'You will learn ADLs. And we are running out of places that will take you.'

'What are ADL's?' I asked.

'Like how to cook and clean – Activities of Daily Living, Alexis.'

'I don't want to learn how to cook or clean. I can't cook.'

'And you learn to clean.'

'I can't clean.'

'Well, there's nowhere else for you, so you're going to have to go there.'

'I'm not going there.'

Dr Hart came again the next day. She said, 'Okay, Alexis, let's talk about rehab. Now, this is what we're going to say to make sure you get in.'

'Felicity, I'm not going.'

Like most placements, you can't go unless you agree to engage. You must want to go. As if anyone actually wants to go. But the alternative was worse, so I stopped saying, 'I don't want to go.'

'Look, Alexis. Think about it. Rehab is in the community. You stay there for up to a year, then you can go home. If you don't take this, you're going to a locked place. They're not going to keep you in here, and they will not discharge you.'

'Well, we'll see about this section, because I have a tribunal in two weeks.'

'Be that as it may, Alexis, this interview is in two days' time. So, just do the interview, do a good job, and then if you go off your section, good. If you don't, at least you're covered.'

'Fine. That's a good idea. Thank you, Felicity. What should I say?' Felicity used to work in rehab. She prepared me. I wrote everything down. This process, as simple as it was, eased anxiety. I hate the unknown.

I did the interview. I nailed all the questions. They said, 'We think you're going to be really suitable for this. It's wonderful you want to develop your activities of daily living, your ADLs.'

'Yeah, I really need to learn to cook for my daughter and do the washing. Actually, I can do the washing. I just can't fold clothes.'

I got into rehab, and I went to my tribunal. I told them, 'Truthfully, I'm not suicidal. I want to go home. I have autism. I'm not mentally ill. There's nothing wrong with me.'

They said I lacked insight into my condition. Because of this I was dangerous. I didn't think I was dangerous and told them so. But because I didn't think I was dangerous, that was why they thought I was dangerous.

They re-sectioned me for six months. I was pissed off. My risk was assumed by people who didn't know my condition or needs.

That doctors misunderstood my niche interest in suicide was documented in the H5 legal document. An H5 is the form doctors use to renew a section. Just one doctor and one form can do this. The power these people hold ...

CHAPTER 47

Rehabilitation

19ᵗʰ October 2015

The deputy ward manager of Oaken, Leroy, drove me to Oxlip Rehab on 19ᵗʰ October. As we were travelling, I realised this was one of a handful of times I had been transferred in a car. Again, I was thinking that this was going be the last place I'd be an inpatient before I went home and got on with my life. I was positive and looking forward to making this work.

Step 1: Get off the section.

I was greeted warmly by a nurse named Dawn and the HCA Janet. It was a genuine warmth, which I had found to be rare in the NHS. I hadn't experienced this for a while and it took me by surprise. The house was large, on the corner of a residential road. Nothing about the outside screamed, 'This is a hospital full of crazy people.' In fact, Leroy had trouble finding it. When he located the correct house, I noticed its garden. The garden was big and I could run in it. What a relief. I was worried that by moving into a house I might not be able to go outside if I didn't have Section 17 leave to leave the premises. I didn't need to worry.

Janet took me upstairs to my new room. It was very big, about five metres by ten metres. I assessed the space – I could do yoga in here. The place was immaculate. Janet told me they had just bought me new bed sheets, white with turquoise and blue butterflies on them. It felt so good to have bed clothes that weren't sanitised or standardised. I felt like a human again. Sectioned but human.

Janet helped me unpack and chatted to me. I was struck by her humanity. She clearly wanted to talk. Nobody had told her to. Janet has incredible shoulder-length, straight silver hair. She explained about the groups I had to attend and gave me a timetable for the week before she left.

After I unpacked, I went downstairs. Leroy had gone. He didn't say goodbye. The time was approaching 3.58pm. The office door was at the bottom of the stairs between the back door to the garden and the front door. As usual it had a glass window. However, this had been constructed in a subtle, normalising way.

I knocked tentatively on the office door. Dawn said, 'Hi, Alexis. You've come for your medication?' Dawn had long, ginger hair she wore down. It was thick, with not a strand of grey. I couldn't take my eyes off it. I told Dawn that her parents were most likely carriers of the mutated MC1R gene to have produced that red hair.

Dawn was about 50 years old. I learnt later that she had two sons my age. One was a zoologist and the other a builder. One of them had red hair so the father must have carried that gene.

'Yeah,' I said in response to her question.

'Come in, come in.'

'What? In the office?'

'Yes, come in. Sit down.' Okay, so this had never happened in an NHS facility. She pointed to a chair right by the medication cabinet. Dawn sat down too. She started talking to me. I was stunned again. She and Janet were the only staff here and they had spent about 30 minutes talking to me today.

I sat with her next to the medicine cabinet. I interrupted her as it was past four o'clock in the afternoon.

'It's 4.01pm now. Can I have that tablet, please?'

'Yes, of course, of course.' She opened the medicine cabinet in front of me. This had not happened either, besides at York. I could not speak as I was still processing what was happening. I thought of how I got here to this lovely place, and silently thanked Dr Felicity Hart.

Dawn popped the tablet out of the packet, and it broke into three pieces. Oh, no. That was a controlled drug so she must account for the broken one in the records. I explained I couldn't take the tablet because it was in three pieces. Dawn didn't listen and continued urging me to take it, explaining that all the pieces were there and the dose would be the same. I couldn't express what was happening. So, I just held the packet. Dawn also was holding the packet.

Dawn said firmly, 'Alexis, give me the packet.' I couldn't let go so pulled the packet from her hand. I stood up gently, knowing that Ritalin is very soft, popped a tablet myself, and swallowed it. Dawn was saying something but all I heard was noise.

I left the room, with my heart pounding in my chest. Every part of my sensory system was activated. Outside the office I took some deep breaths. I could hear Dawn say to Janet, 'This isn't going to last long. Not a good start.' Dawn didn't know I have super hearing when I'm overloaded. Although Leroy would have "handed over" to her, I doubt he talked about overload and meltdown.

I melted down, wandered in the road and was brought back by the police. I kept thinking, *Where do I fit in this world?* I didn't want to leave here so soon. I was delighted with how things had started. I was so angry with myself for the way I dealt with that situation and struggled to analyse how I could have improved the interaction. Remembering the time I was transferred from

PICU to Clover, and then four hours later from Clover to PICU, I decided to go back and speak to Dawn. I didn't want her to phone Oaken and tell them to come and get me.

I knocked on the office door. Dawn told me I didn't need to knock. She said, 'Alexis, do you drink tea?' I told her I did and said I didn't want tea, but I wanted to talk to her. Dawn explained that tea is very helpful. She proceeded to make me a cup of piping hot tea in a porcelain mug. We talked, and for the first time since York I drank from a vessel that wasn't made of plastic.

Dawn showed interest when I talked. And we sat in the office with the door closed. Obviously, she wasn't of the opinion I was about to pounce on her. She focused on what I was saying and asked questions. Not once did she make a recommendation for better behaviour, and I felt no judgement. Dawn showed respect, understanding, and refrained from suggestions or counter arguments. She just listened. I was so grateful. I thought that I would get well here. I wasn't sure I was sick but voicing such statements wasn't helpful. During our discussion I, too, learnt a few things.

I had now been in rehab about six hours. In that time, I had seen just a few people walking past the office window. There were seven other distressed people in the building, yet it was quiet and peaceful. I asked to go out. Janet took me for a walk and we went to the park. It was a short walk from the house. Janet had lived in the area all her life. She told me that in a week or so I could go to the beach, a 10-minute walk.

I didn't attend the afternoon group that day. But I was expected to attend the following day. Actually, I wanted to attend, if a little nervous about it. From Monday to Friday, there were two groups. And there was morning and evening cleaning. Janet told me this during our walk.

I asked what time dinner was. Janet smiled at me and I watched her mouth. Dinner was when I cooked it.

I knew none of these nurses. I'd known all the nurses at PICU and the acute units for years. My social skills were being tested. I could see that staff in Oxlip had a good relationship with people. Each person stayed an average of a year, so they knew each other well. I was breaking in as the new person and I was welcome.

That evening, I ate Weetabix I bought from the supermarket with Janet. I slept well that night.

*

I was up early as usual and went for a run to the park. This wasn't questioned. All I was asked was whether I felt okay for a run. I came back, had a shower, and got my own breakfast. More Weetabix.

The morning meeting started at nine o'clock in the morning sharp. Nobody was late. I said 'Hello' to everyone. Jobs were allocated for the week. We all had our ADLs. They included:

Cleaning kitchen surfaces, emptying the dust bin, and washing up

Cleaning the kitchen floor

Cleaning living-room floor

Cleaning the landing

Cleaning the calming room

Cleaning the dining room

There was a job for each of us. I'd never done cleaning before, really, or cooking, shopping, or budgeting, because I always had money and lived overseas. I'd had a maid.

We were well supported in our tasks if we needed help, which I did. Over the coming months I didn't seem to get any better at the jobs to staff's frustration.

In school, you get thousands of chances to learn. You repeat and repeat. But you don't get this luxury with cleaning, dressing, washing, ironing, shopping, and cooking. You might be shown a handful of times. Then you're expected to know how to do it. I was given far more opportunities to learn academics and sports than functional ADL skills. Think about this. If someone showed me once a week how to clean the living-room floor, it would take me 15 years to get 1,000 opportunities to learn. Once a week was too spread out. I wasn't able to pick up the skills.

Now nobody would do it for me. This was apparently what rehab is all about. I had to go out shopping – otherwise I would have no food. At first, I only ate cereal. However, as things calmed down and my spoons replenished, I became more capable. I met with Courtenay, the OT. I would be seeing her every week on Wednesday, and I told her I thought I needed a standardised meal plan. She was taken aback. Courtenay did not know about autism. I found myself in the position of explaining something I didn't fully understand myself.

I told Courtenay I couldn't *put together* the skills needed for shopping. I could walk to the shop. I could make a list. I could find an item. I could carry money in my pocket. I could calculate the correct money. But stringing together those different tasks was too hard. Courtenay found this hard to believe.

We went shopping together. Courtenay saw there were so many nuances of decisions and actions in these tasks. My phobia of fruit was a big challenge in a supermarket. In every market when you walk in there are the fruit and veg. And all that fruit is moving around in people's trolleys.

Courtenay the OT, Dr Mitchell the psychologist, and I sat and explored strategies in case a problem arose. The stakes were high so I was anxious, which made shopping even more of a challenge. If I failed and something went wrong, I would be sent back to acute, or worse, PICU. I could now see I needed rehab.

Dr Mitchell was a good woman. She spelt out the nuances to me. She worked with the staff closely and together we went through the cues and skills for shopping. For example, 'I need to go shopping. I don't have X, Y, and Z. X, Y, and Z cost 10 pounds. They are on the left of the supermarket. Let's look at my schedule. On Friday morning after group I can go to the store. I must bring my ATM card.'

Never in my life would I have thought I needed this level of support, but at this time I did. I couldn't function without it.

The next shift, Lisa, an HCA, and I worked on a shopping list. But when the list was complete I said to her, 'I just can't go shopping, Lisa.'

She said, 'Of course you can. It's easy, Lexi.'

I said, 'No, it's too stressful, and I don't want to walk past the fruit. I've never done any shopping like this before.' I'd always bought whatever the hell I liked. Now I had to budget. I had 26 pounds a week. That was nothing. I could have spent that in two minutes. When I worked, I would eat out all the time, because I was overseas and it was cheap. I didn't have to worry about money because there was just me. I had a good salary and was in a developing country. And before that, when I was swimming, the National Performance Centre looked after me.

Lisa said, 'You can use a standardised meal plan.'

'I don't know how to cook.'

Lisa reassured me. So did Dawn and all the other staff. I had my meal plan, and a list of ingredients. I didn't know how my mouth would respond to this food, because I felt different every day. I was still so overloaded that if the food had a strong taste or smell, I could not eat it. But staff insisted that I wasn't going to spend a year just living on Weetabix. Because they cared about me, I trusted them. Gradually, with support, I learnt a new meal every few days. The staff would cook it with me using a basic cookbook.

I made everything from scratch because I had to know the ingredients were healthy. I used no sauces. I'm vegetarian. If I had a veggie burger, I had to make it myself. So, when I was doing my OT, it was all cooking for 10 weeks. Sometimes, I would accidently set the pan on fire. But here mistakes were allowed.

Rehab was the place where I realised I wouldn't be good at certain things. I learnt that despite my best efforts I might still fail. This was okay. I admitted to Dr Mitchell, Nurse Ethel, and many nurses that I was stuck. I didn't know what to do. They had no experience in autism, but together we tried hard to get solutions. And I faced my fears alongside caring professionals. For many problems like the ADLs, resources and solutions appeared. For other problems, I searched and came up with nothing, but I learnt to tell my truth.

I had spent a long time covering up my mistakes and being embarrassed about myself. Indeed, I now had spent years being "treated" for being myself. I wished for a handy mistake eraser to cover up my flaws, and a time machine to take me back to pre-meltdown. Now I was being honest about my failures with nurses and HCAs. The people here listened, and I could expose myself safely. I guess I had little choice, but there was something liberating about failing in front of others. Their perspectives were a mirror. I felt that staff saw me for the first time, and I saw me for the first time. It was like I was being born again. I didn't have to waste energy and spoons by covering myself. I let go of embarrassment, shame and blame, and concentrated on learning and growing.

I was cooking quite a few meals on my own. One day, however, there was a flame in the frying pan higher than my head. It was a real scare. Neo, the peer support worker, put the flame out with a fire extinguisher. I realised I wasn't yet ready for anything complex and unsupervised.

I had more spoons available now that my executive functioning was better. When you cook, there are many things you must think about at the same time. When I'd done it repeatedly, using a simple flowchart, I could succeed. I also had a safety checklist I would go through before every meal. This was progress.

I learnt later that Dr Malvada, the responsible clinician, had added "arson" to my risk assessment.

CHAPTER 48

Learning to Manage

November 2015

Night was a time of stress and worry because I would experience flashbacks. These always came with no warning. I had them before and they increased since I arrived at rehab. I think it's because my brain was more relaxed so I wasn't always on high alert.

The most frequent flashbacks were of seclusion. These usually happened when I was cold. I would wake up feeling like I was in the freezing 136 suite. I'd remember the awful cold, the eyes of staff watching me and how I'd begged them. Mostly it was an overwhelming sense of desperation.

I would flash back when I heard keys jingling. Suddenly I was filled with anxiety. I'd be back in Ivy seclusion with staff getting closer to the door, with me thinking, *I'm getting out now*. Then the sound would fade away. This intense flashback lasted seconds, but was like an hour of panic. It was special torture for me because of my need for predictability.

With Dr Mitchell I developed a routine to manage these. Communication between nurses and HCAs was excellent, so everyone supported the routine. I would go downstairs, make a cup of tea, and sit with the night staff in silence. After about

45 minutes I had calmed enough to go back upstairs. The staff would say, 'Good night, Alexis.'

Compared to an acute unit, rehab was not a busy place. There were few people, and everyone was chilled so there was no kicking off. I was bored. There wasn't anyone to hang out with since most residents stayed in their rooms. I went home at weekends. Abi's school was 10 minutes from the rehab, so I picked her up and dropped her off every day. I had routine, but aside from ADLs and groups, I was lonely.

I first got to know Michael because he would always sit across from me in the morning meeting. He had a diagnosis of bipolar disorder. He was a very intelligent and creative guy who sometimes experienced extreme states of being.

I learnt from Michael that most people in rehab are not sectioned. The idea is to get them back to the community. Michael, like me, didn't think he was ill. He explained that the best thing to do is agree that you are ill so you're seen as having insight. My phone wasn't working properly, which led him to disclose that he used to work for Apple. We shared how we came to be viewed as "mental", and spent hours discussing what illness was.

Michael and I went for walks into town and had a coffee now and again. We discussed iatrogenic effects of psychiatric life. Harm is common. I hadn't realised it. The profession doesn't like to admit it, but when you scratch beneath the shiny veneer of somewhere like rehab, it's there to see.

One day we had an interesting dialogue with Sarah, a nurse. She's an advocate for the imbalance theory of illness and believes in the efficacy of drugs. We strongly challenged her position. She was willing to debate her medical model of depression against our "suffering is part of life" stance.

I made the point that, 'With more advances in technology, neuroscience, and treatments, more people are sicker to the extent that they are disabled, need government handouts, and are addicted to meds.'

Michael backed me up with, 'We are not saying drugs don't help some people. We have been inside for years. We know they help. But what we are saying is that they cause more harm than good for the majority.'

I added a follow-up punch, 'The chemical imbalance theory is a fallacy, Sarah. The only chemical imbalance that occurs in your brain is the one that happens as a result of taking the drug.' I'm pretty sure we didn't change her thinking, but I enjoyed the discussion. It was good banter and stimulating.

I realised that I liked people, but I wasn't good at talking and making friends. Yes, the nurses and I had fun playing Scrabble and Bananagrams. However, this wasn't the way forward. Playing board games passed the time, but it wasn't rehabilitating me.

The groups were rather peculiar at Oxlip. They didn't focus on anything useful. For example, each week I was there the groups were the same and involved the following activities.

Playing Pictionary: I hated the group and it made me upset. After the first few weeks, I didn't have to go. I found that I looked like an idiot. For example, imagine the word is "pizza". The person drawing does a circle with smaller circles in it. I don't see a pizza. I just see what it is. I can't imagine what it might be if it's not that thing. I was forced to articulate my guesses because of the size of teams, and people would laugh.

Walk and Talk: where you go for a walk and have a chat. This usually ended with us sitting in a coffee shop.

Out and About: we chose a destination where we had to take public transport to get there.

Current Affairs: we read tabloids.

Art and Crafts: we did colouring or made things. As I progressed I did sewing work with two HCAs, Betsy and Lisa.

Mental Health Awareness: this is where the pseudoscience was used to brainwash us into thinking we were ill and into accepting "treatment" that probably wasn't needed.

There was a lot of time between groups. Often when the unit was quiet and people were at home with their families, ginger Dawn would take me for hot chocolate to Costa or Nero's. This reminded me of being at work and nipping out with a colleague. We would chat about normal stuff, not illness, not bloody mental health, not autism. Dawn was into cross-stitch, and she taught me. I'm very good at it now. We would sit together in the TV room, pick a pattern and work out cool colour schemes. I learnt quickly and enjoyed mastering it.

HCA Betsy taught me to sew and Lisa taught me to crochet. I made a beautiful mermaid tail for Abi. Learning ADLs gave me a feeling of accomplishment. It was also relaxing. Whenever I felt stressed or a bit anxious, I would sit and do needlework.

Sport was still a big need for me. A guy called Chester was the Occupational Therapy Technical Instructor, OTTI. He was a very cool man who played the guitar. He had an earring that stretched his ear. Chester was very active and down to earth. I joined a local gym close to rehab. Chester and I would play badminton there and also table tennis once a week. I worked out for an hour a day at the gym. I did lots of weights and this satisfied my sensory needs. I didn't need to spin and roll around the place, as my vestibular system and proprioceptive system were finally content.

A few times when the very sensitive fire alarms went off in rehab, I fled. We planned a running route so if anything happened to me, they would know which route I was on. Chester helped me persuade staff to allow me to join a running group. It was a community-based running club set up as a charity in memory of a young child who had died from cancer. I ran with the group twice a week and made a lot of friends. Then I started running distance with them. I built up to running a half marathon in just two months.

CHAPTER 49

What Xmas Means to Me

24ᵗʰ December 2015

I'd had staff help now for three months. The multidisciplinary team thought I needed to shop on my own. Dr Malvada said she would think about removing my section if I was more successful with "normal" activities.

Neo, the peer support worker employed to relate to us because she had been in the system, would take us out for walks. She attached herself to my hip because my road awareness was still iffy. I was trying to work on this among all the other things.

On a Monday after ward round, I went shopping. I was anxious but determined. I wasn't overloaded and the roads were not an issue. I had also learnt where items were in the shop, so my process was quicker. In the early days, staff would say, 'Alexis, just get the beans.' I'd then get stuck on details, unable to scan.

I'd say, 'I can see all these patterns that you can't see, but I can't see the beans.' These days, however, I knew where stuff was.

Staff and I hadn't accounted for the Xmas change-the-store-about routine. Though frustrated by these changes, I still believed in myself. I wasn't about to admit defeat. That ableist voice in my head told me I should be able to do it.

This was the one time a member of staff wasn't with me. There I was standing in the middle of the aisle, looking at the myriad cans on the shelf. There was Christmas music playing, making it hard to concentrate. I had just walked through the fruit and veg aisle. The holiday shoppers were weaving their rattling trolleys in no particular direction. Kids were running around, people greeting each other, chatting, and brushing past me.

Just don't touch me. It hurts. Plus the bright lights are all red and green because it's Christmas.

I was trying to find this tin of chickpeas. They had moved them and I didn't know what aisle to look in. Anxiety crept in.

I was looking and looking. Okay, I scanned along, then went down the shelf, scanned along. I couldn't just look at the whole thing. I saw individual things. This is called local processing. Most people see global process. This means seeing the "big picture". It's like this picture. I don't see the whole shape (global). I see the individual small letters (local) first. And I count them. It's instinctual.

```
BBBBBBBBBBBB   MMMMMMMMM   PPPPP        PPPPP    SSSSS       SSSS
BBBBBBBBBBBB   MMMMMMMM    PPPP         PPPP     SSSSS       SSSS
BBBB           MMM         PPPP         PPPP     SSSSS       SSSS
BBBB           MMM         PPPP      PPPP        SSSSS    SSSS
BBBBBBBBBBB    MMM         PPPP    PPPP          SSSSS SSSS
BBBBBBBBBBB    MMMMMMMM    PPPP  PPPP            SSSSS SSSSS
BBBB           MMMMMMMM       PPPP PPPP          SSSSS    SSSSS
BBBB           MMM           PPPPPPP             SSSSS       SSSSS
BBBB           MMM            PPPPP              SSSSS       SSSSS
BBBBBBBBBBBB   MMM             PPPP              SSSSS        SSSSS
BBBBBBBBBBBB   MMM              PP               SSSSS         SSSSS
```

So, I was looking, and it was taking ages. I was getting more and more stressed because I couldn't find the tin. I had to succeed. I didn't want to mess up. I wanted to be off section. This was the kind of thing I needed to do. Dr Malvada told me so. Due to the stress, I didn't recognise that I was becoming overloaded.

Then this shop assistant came along with a police officer. They asked me, 'Can we help you?'

I said, 'No, thank you.'

They came back later and asked again. By this time, I couldn't speak, so I just looked at them. They went away. Thank goodness. Okay, I just needed to find this one item and leave.

Suddenly more police showed up. Rehab staff had encouraged me to wear a wrist band that said Alexis Quinn, Autism, with Oxlip's phone number on it. I showed them this wrist band, thinking, please don't handcuff me. Anyway, they did handcuff me because I didn't want to leave my task of shopping unfinished. They took me to Oxlip.

Rehab staff followed the usual routine after an arrest. I was given tablets, calmed in the calming room and debriefed. I was denied unescorted Section 17 leave for a while.

I saw Dr Malvada the following Monday after the incident. I had to see her every week because I was on section. 'Tell, me Alexis, what happened this time? Because it seems you are not making progress again. You are stepping backwards every time you are given responsibility. Are you avoiding it? Why is that?'

Wow, too many questions. I had asked her not to do that. I responded to the last question.

'Well, doctor, I now know why I can't find an item in the store. I believe it is because I have an innate preference for local processing. This precipitated the event. Perhaps you could tell me how to train my visual perception. Then it probably won't happen again.'

'What on earth does that have to do with being arrested? Alexis, if you want to come off section then you need to stop getting yourself into trouble.'

'Yes, I know that. I agree. I'm asking you how to better globally process information. Did you cover that in medical school? I want to know how to integrate piecemeal information into a coherent whole. If I could do this, then I'd be able to locate items better in the supermarket. It is possible. I've read about it.'

'Alexis, I just wish that you would learn to manage. You need to stop having what you call "meltdowns". That's all. It's simple. Can you agree to that?'

'No, I can't. If it was simple I would have done it already. Don't patronise me. And meltdowns are a term used by the autism community. I didn't make the word up. If you read even a little on autism then you would know about meltdowns.'

'I don't need to read, Alexis. I know what I am saying.'

'Thank goodness you know what you are doing. For a minute, I thought you were clueless about processing. Tell me, how can I combine information about objects, like chickpeas and their surroundings, to understand scenes? What exercise can I do?'

'Actually, Alexis, the problem is that you are ill. You don't seem to grasp that.'

I ignored her ignorant statement. I felt like I was going around in circles. She wasn't listening to a suggestion that would actually help! Was she stupid? I decided to meet her halfway.

'I would like you to get me speech and language training. My receptive language is underdeveloped, as you know. If this improved, then so would my global processing knowledge. Then I could use words and their syntax to understand sentences and social cues, including context. This would mean I could understand interactions between people. This will reduce overload and meltdown. What do you think of the suggestion?'

'I think that you keep deflecting the real issue. You are dangerous to yourself and others and until you get that under control I can't help you.'

'No, Dr Malvada, I am not. We have been over this. I understand you are frustrated by my recent incident in the supermarket. I am too. It was awful being handcuffed and basically assaulted for no reason. I am trying to tell you–'

She cut me off. 'There you go again, Alexis, shifting the blame onto someone else. You must take responsibility. Manage your emotions better and use your words properly to communicate. Don't ignore people when they are trying to talk to you'.

I was getting angry. Think about it. There I am in the supermarket and just because I wasn't talking, they arrested me. Why? I wasn't doing anything. I was just looking for the fucking chickpeas. They thought I was on drugs. Now I was really annoyed.

'Actually, the incident happened because people don't tolerate difference. They didn't like my "weak central coherence", or inability to see "the big picture". I was stuck looking. I was searching, focused on the detail.'

'Well, why didn't you tell them that then?' Malvada probed.

'Of course I told them. They didn't listen. And then I was stressed and became overloaded.' Ahhhh … I was frustrated. I took a deep breath. 'Doctor, in order for this interaction to be of any use to either of us, please understand that successful interaction for me with the world requires both local and global processing. There are so many behavioural goals you have for me that could be met if you would just help. Can we agree on that?'

'Okay, Alexis. We are done for today. You don't demand things from me and tell me how to do my job. If you don't want my advice, that is fine. But you will remain on section.'

'Fucking hell. You are an idiot! I have just told you that I want your help. I want to know how to attend to information. I want to know how to look at things as a whole. I am not choosing not to process, you idiot. It isn't a choice. The two are different, with importantly different implications for remediation. Can you help with that or not?'

'I'll see you next week, Alexis. Try to have a better week.'

'Thanks, doctor. This interaction has helped zero. Try to listen to your next patient.'

*

Interestingly, social and communication issues affect executive function ability as well! If you don't understand context, that undermines executive function. If you don't understand what someone has just said, that weakens executive function. Another dot had just been connected. But the clinical psychologist on the learning disability team couldn't help me because she wasn't in the mental health team. And Dr Malvada clearly wasn't interested.

So, I needed to sort out my processing and executive function problems. Rehab staff didn't know where to start. I read a good analogy about executive function which calmed my frustrations about my high intelligence yet poor performance at ADLs. It's like a computer that works great, good programming and good files and software but the output device is compromised. The printer isn't working and the monitor is flickering. This settled me down. I wasn't stupid, lazy, or crazy. I am capable. I just need the right means for output. This was helpful. I could work on it myself.

CHAPTER 50

At University, Still Mad

25th January to early February 2016

I was going to university now. I had passed my counselling skills course at college. I had been advised to do this course by a member of staff in Falton Green to improve my communication. It helped my listening skills a lot. Now I was studying psychology at an evening course in the city, researching and learning some complicated topics.

It was a constant source of frustration to me and staff, mostly Dr Malvada, that I was intelligent but lacked ability in basic functional areas. After months of trying I still couldn't master my ADLs. I understood it was important. I couldn't do the simple things that everyone in the world can do when they're 10. But I was going to university.

Getting to university was an issue. I was arrested once when Chester asked me to take the train. It was awful. And every time I failed, I was a step closer to being transferred to acute. Dr Malvada was losing patience. I told her time and again I didn't need a cure. I didn't expect her and her medicine to help me.

'Alexis,' she would say, 'it is my job.'

'No, it isn't,' I'd argue. 'You are colluding with the standardised, overly technical, and overextended psychiatry model that is prevalent, but actually doesn't work. Don't treat me like that. It has hurt me in the past and it hurts me now. Let's be practical.'

'I am practical, Alexis. You need to decrease your emotional liability and stop kicking off.' This was in response to me being detained at the train station.

'You need to understand that I don't feel emotions. I need emotional education. I need healing with Dr Mitchell using the interplay of autism, my context and history. You are causing more harm because you not considering these things. You assume that because I am academically clever, I am also emotionally intelligent and have great ADLs. Do you understand that?'

'Yes, and right now I want you to stop reacting the way you do to the fire alarm. I want you to be more road-aware. I want you to be more social and stop kicking off. We are done for the week. See you next week. I expect to hear that you have successfully completed your ADLs.'

Dr Mitchell introduced me to Dr Carrie, specialist in charge of the autism unit for Kingshire and Heysham. Dr Carrie told me that many autistics do not progress well with ADLs because of executive functioning problems. My issues clearly.

CHAPTER 51

Jenny and David

One weekend my mum planned a visit from our former neighbour, Jenny, whom I hadn't seen for years. She moved away when I was about 10. She and her partner David, a retired doctor, were coming to visit. I didn't know him, and I didn't want to see Jenny.

I said, 'Mum, I'm just not going to come home. I'll stay at Oxlip.'

She said, 'Lexi, that's ridiculous. Of course, you're coming home.'

'Look, I really don't want to see them. I hate socialising and the conversation will start with, "So, what are you doing these days, Lexi?" I will end up being a self-narrating zoo exhibit. I don't want to talk about myself or my problems and I don't want to sit at a table. Can't you have the dinner party when I'm not here?'

'No, Lexi. We're not changing our life for you. You need to socialise.'

'Well, I don't need to.'

'Then just go out with Daya.' Daya and I have been friends since I was born. She is like a sister. We lived opposite each other in Morecombe Cove.

'Okay. That's a good idea.' So, I did go home, and Abi, my friend Daya, and I went out. We had a big day out, for four-

and-a-half hours. I thought, *There's no way they will still be in the house when I get home.* But there they were when I opened the door.

I said, 'Oh, hello.' I was imagining the conversation they'd been having before I came in. What's Thomas doing? My parents would say, well, Thomas is the world champion rower, has a job in London, and he's happily married. Then it would be, what's Alexis doing? They would say, oh, Alexis is a mental patient. She's had a breakdown.

This happened often. When Josh was young, people would ask, 'What's Alexis up to?'

My parents would say, 'Alexis is a straight-A student, and is swimming for Britain. Thomas is living in Australia. Oh, Josh is just … Josh.'

I walked in, and they asked, 'How are you?'

Fuck off, it's none of your business.

What am I supposed to say? I guess something like 'I am fine, thank you.' I got my tea and was heading upstairs.

Jenny said, 'Come sit down, Lexi. Have some cheese and biscuits.'

'Oh, no, thanks,' I said. 'I just had dinner, actually. I don't need any cheese and biscuits.' I felt a little bad. 'Well, I will, but I have to put Abi to bed in a minute.' So, there I was having this chat. Jenny, but especially David, was asking me about everything.

I said, 'You know what? I will tell you. I'm going to tell you what it's like.' David was a retired doctor, a GP, so he was interested in hearing about my experience. I told them everything from the day Josh died to the present time, every incident, admission, and drug.

David was shocked. I don't think he quite believed me. He kept questioning me. He told me I seemed intelligent. I didn't look mental, nor did I sound mental. He wanted to understand,

and to see my complaints and the NHS Trust's responses. We chatted for a few more hours.

In the end, both David and Jenny knew everything. They both wanted to help me.

I said, 'I doubt it. I'm sectioned and the doctor isn't pleased with my progress. In fact, she keeps talking about escalating the service if I don't improve.'

'What? That's ridiculous. I can't detect any problem with you, aside from that caused by the restrictive practice that that doctor puts on you,' David said.

'A place more secure than an acute ward I think. I am sometimes a problem. I can't do quite a few things. I'll admit that much. I'm currently not able in many areas.'

'Nor would I be, Lex, in your circumstance,' said Jenny. 'What we should do is, I'll just kidnap you. You can come and live with us.' She laughed, but I didn't find it very funny.

I said, 'No, I don't think that will work. It's illegal, first of all, for you to kidnap me.' This wasn't because I didn't want to be kidnapped. It's actually illegal to take somebody who's on a section for longer than the Section 17 leave allows, and out of a 50-mile radius from the rehab house.

Jenny smiled at my musings – turned out she was joking.

After this, Jenny and David got involved. I spoke with them on the phone and they came to visit me a few times in rehab. They got to see the restrictions and control, how I was contained. But I told them I was lucky. Rehab is open. There are doors I can walk out of. And the staff are pleasant and caring.

David wasn't much focused on the staff. He was more interested in the doctor, who he called a "lazy woman". He argued that Dr Malvada was lazy because she displayed behaviour that showed a lack of good sense and judgement.

'She must be intelligent and hard-working, David. She's a doctor.'

'She might be, Lex, but she isn't demonstrating a humanity in her approach to you. I think you have asthma from the SSRIs. Have you considered that?'

'No. I never had asthma before, but I didn't know it was caused by SSRIs.'

'Polypharmacy, the mixing of meds, is not a good thing. I am not happy with the cocktail you're taking, especially when you have nothing to treat. Your symptoms are a response to your environment. And you are not suicidal. You just need a heart-centred and non-pathologising approach.'

'She ignores what I say. It's like I'm not sitting in front of her. It's more than even the failure of imagination in most of the psychiatrists' interpretations of me.'

'She is scared of you,' David said.

'No, I don't believe that. She has enormous power over me, that's for sure. And she expects deference from not just me, but also the lovely rehab staff. I've seen her take it as impertinence if my ideas challenge hers. The only person she does listen to is Dr Mitchell.'

Over the following months, David tried to further demystify the aura of self-serving legitimacy he believed Malvada was demonstrating. He looked her up and did his research on autism. He and Jenny attended an autism workshop in London to learn more. He came to agree that I have autism and nothing more than contextual despair born out of my situation.

David and Jenny looked into the law to challenge Malvada and the psychiatric practice I had fallen to. I was coming around to David's way of thinking. Every week when I sat with Dr Malvada, I noticed her inherent stupidity of blindly adhering to a failed theory and practice when treating me.

*

When my mum and dad went on holiday, David and Jenny invited me to stay in their home. As my family was away, I was granted leave to Jenny's house only. It was a little over 50 miles from the rehab, and the special leave was written up by Dr Malvada. We had a nice first evening. David quizzed me on autism and what was happening, but aside from that I enjoyed the peace and quiet, and the normalcy of a family home without pictures of Josh all around and memories to contend with.

The next day Jenny said she would take me to London. I told her this wasn't allowed. She said, 'They won't know.'

'Yes, but it's illegal. I don't have leave for London. My leave is only for Red Rake Bay, Morecombe Cove, and your house.'

Jenny said, 'We're going into London. I'll get tickets for a show.'

I said, 'Mate, we can't. First, I can't go on a train.'

She said, 'Yes, you can.'

So, on 13th February, we got on the train. This was nerve-wracking, but I was with Jenny. When I went with Chester to university it had been okay, and I told myself that this was no different. We went to London and watched the West End play *Red Velvet* on Charing Cross Road. I really enjoyed the show. Nobody inside the theatre knew I was mental. I was like any other person. Theatre provided a much-needed boost. I thanked Jenny again and again.

When we got back to their house, I was more myself than I'd been in a long time. I hadn't been to a play since before Josh died.

Jenny said, 'I'm going to kidnap you. You can live here.' Logistically there was plenty of space in their house and they had a large garden and a lake. It looked like a nature reserve. However, being kidnapped wouldn't solve my problems. I needed to work through them. I politely declined and we kept in touch. David often called me and gave me advice. He told me under no circumstances should I discuss suicide with Dr Malvada.

He schooled me on mind blindness. 'Individuals that are normal have an unfathomable yet ubiquitous ability to mind read. Because you don't have this ability, you are shooting yourself in the foot, Lexi.'

'Actually, I am normal. I am just neurodivergent.'

'Whatever you want to call yourself, you don't understand ordinary social interactions. Normal people behave as if they have an implicit theory of mind, and this allows them to explain and predict others' behaviour in terms of their presumed thoughts and feelings. So, tell me, why is Dr Malvada continuing to section you?'

'I have no idea.'

'I do. I know why.'

'You've never met her.'

'No, but I can read her mind.'

'Really?'

'Yes. She thinks you are suicidal.'

'I am not. I've told her that.'

'Yes, but she thinks you are because you're researching it in detail. She believes that to keep you safe she has to control you.'

'She doesn't need to control me. I am not suicidal.'

'I know that, Lexi. I've been a doctor for 30 years. I know. But she is naive and nervous of you. You are a six-foot tall, clever, athletic woman who talks incessantly about suicide. What do you expect her to think?'

'I don't know. I expect her to realise it's an interest.'

'You see, without mentalising, you are not realising that she's coming up with an outlandish interpretation of your research interests. I know it's because she is not listening. But you are not mentalising. You are effectively winding each other up!'

'I see. What you're saying is that by interpreting others' behaviour, we automatically take account of their mental state, their desires, and their beliefs. I am failing to do this.'

'Precisely.'

I was immensely grateful to David for that. I had learnt a lot.

*

After my stay in their house, David wanted me off section and back in the community. Both David and Jenny told me they would do whatever they could to make it happen. I had never looked at my situation like they did. I thought I was faulty, but now I had more self-belief. In three years, almost no one had called me smart or listened to me. I had little confidence, but I was sure from my research I wasn't ill. Couldn't I stay in rehab voluntarily? The doors were open, so what difference did it make? I could do more "therapy" off section.

CHAPTER 52

Communication

Dr Mitchell came every week. I had a psychology session with her on Wednesdays and saw her on Mondays in ward round. During psychology, we worked through immediate issues like changes in environment, managing my new pseudo-freedom, creating routines, and identifying overload. We went over any incidents I had had and, crucially, we prepped for ward round.

One important thing she did was help me communicate with Dr Malvada, who had no knowledge of autism and did not try to educate herself. As my friend David suggested, I found she did indeed lack good sense and judgement. Dr Malvada was parsimonious in the empathy she would show. She remained clinically detached. Dr Mitchell was the bridge between us.

Dr Malvada was what you would call long-winded. Conversations were circular, 'Well, this happened last week, and we need to think about this, and we don't know if you're going to be able to do that. I'd like to give you more leave, you know that, but I'm just not sure.'

When she got to the end, I would ask, 'So, what's the answer? Can I have more leave or not? I don't know what you've just said.'

No member of staff initially knew know how to talk with me. Dr Mitchell, Dr Carrie, and I helped them to help me. Together we worked through my speech and language report and followed the very clear and concise recommendations.

These included:

UNDERSTANDING OF LANGUAGE	
Communication Style	**Notes**
Provide new information in a written format.	Alexis struggles to process information. Having information written down will help Alexis to retain and process information.
Check that Alexis has understood when presenting her with new information. This should not be simply to ask her if she understands, but by asking her to explain in her own words what she understands.	Her ability to retain information is impaired.
Avoid using complex sentence structures and negative sentences, such as, 'the man is not sitting.' Use simple positive sentence structures, for example, 'the man is standing.'	Alexis struggles to comprehend a range of complex sentence structures.

SOCIAL INTERACTION	
Communication Style	**Notes**
Provide Alexis with feedback with regard to her social skills.	If Alexis uses appropriate social skills, provide her with positive feedback. For example, if Alexis initiates a conversation appropriately by using eye contact or a social convention, give her praise.
Use concrete language and avoid using sarcasm.	Alexis has difficulty understanding sarcasm and non-literal language. She may misinterpret the sarcastic comments and take them literally.
Alexis may misinterpret facial expressions and non-verbal communication. Be clear and concise when explaining something to Alexis and do not rely on your non-verbal communication to convey meaning.	Alexis will struggle to interpret non-verbal communication such as facial expressions, gestures, and body language.

Speech and Language Therapist, Falton Green Therapeutic Campus

Dr Malvada wasn't reasonable. She lectured and blindly inflicted medical interventions. For example, I questioned her on my asthma. She dismissed it. It was this that helped me catch on. Asthma is serious. I could no longer run without an inhaler. How could she ignore that?

David had warned me that this was what she was doing. Even though I had been a successful professional person, Dr Malvada proclaimed that my illness was lifelong, and set about hope-killing in a way that degraded my identity and potential.

I could communicate with nurses and HCAs just fine. Why? Because they accommodated me. Not so with Dr Malvada, but because of her position she was the very person with whom I needed clarity.

CHAPTER 53

My Letter to Dr Malvada

1st February 2016

So, in a desperate attempt to just "try harder" – as Dr Malvada said – I wrote to her prior to the ward round on Monday.

Dear Dr Malvada,

I have realised that I cannot verbally communicate with you effectively. You are confusing and I get frustrated when I can't understand you. This results in my brain processing information more slowly and then I take too long to reply, by which time you have likely talked over me. And the process starts again. This is a problem because I have few forms of release – especially emotional release. Talking is very important because it builds relationships and I want to have a good one with you.

You know what else is difficult? You don't because I haven't told you ... but ... in ward round I often must try to explain and express thoughts, feelings, and emotions I don't understand, and they don't come out of me correctly or you cut me off; in addition I recognise only four emotions. It's hard to explain to you when I don't understand it myself. I suppose it is like asking a child to explain quantum physics or string theory with relation to time travel within the Einsteinian universe.

This is like my problem. But I have a solution. I am writing to you everything I think I need you to know.

I am doing much better here at rehab. However, no matter how often you tell me differently, it is simply impossible to influence my Autistic Spectrum Disorder (though it is possible to change how I exist as a person with ASD), and it is perfectly possible to influence the environment. That is what needs to be focused on. Please, please focus on this. Why don't you?

It is the elusive concept of a "normal" world I am expected to fit into and I want to, but with the environment being so alien, so distressingly chaotic and unreasonable, is it any wonder I have ended up with severe mental ill health? It is the neurotypical way of existing and doing things that is expected. You're asking me to change, to reduce risk by simply trying harder – it's like asking someone with an arm missing to catch a ball with two hands – 'Just try harder – use both hands.' You have said more than once, more than twice, that you don't believe it is a neurological problem. This is harmful because you are essentially blaming me for being me.

The most basic principle and yet one which has yet to be embedded in your psyche is this: forcing me to reside in a neuro-typical rehab without making changes or considering my difference is harmful. And makes me worse. The nurses and support staff don't do this, so why do you?

Every single day, situations arise which clarify the negative effects mental health services' way of doing things have on me. I have been ill-treated for far too long.

So, I need you to understand: I can't keep doing this. My resolve is diminishing. Because time after time, I am essentially told by you that the fault is mine. You say I am the one who needs to change and adapt to the situation, and I am the one who needs to take responsibility for making those adaptations. I feel like you give no thought to how you expect me to do this. Aside from the ineffectual aspect of following this pathway, it is unethical when in the Mental Health Code of Practice you are supposed to make "reasonable adjustment". So, is continuing in this way professionally ethical? Is it appropriate? Is it the way forward in reducing mental ill health? I hope you answer with a resounding NO.

You are looking at me through the wrong lens – I believe you look and think, What is wrong with Alexis? How can we fix her? Rather than Let's see how we can help Alexis to manage her environment as an autistic. *Have a look at the diagnostic criteria to see what I mean. Your approach is unhealthy and, I would argue, unjust; simply because I think differently to most doesn't make me "wrong". I can't change – I'm wired differently to you, whether you like it or not.*

Finally, at some point you need to recognise that your use of language (or perhaps I should say your misuse of language) can have severe and lasting effects. From irksome tautological language in ward round to blatant lies in tribunal reports, I face a barrage of inaccurate and misleading communications. Do you expect me to be okay with that? To deal with it? I can't, and it leads to problematic encounters, that lead to stress, anxiety, and depression. The nurses and support staff have made relatively simple changes which make an enormous difference. Can you do the same, please?

It can work here at rehab. I know it can because of the outstanding progress I have already made. But you scare me. I am petrified of you. Please listen and give me a chance.

Alexis Makenna Quinn

I sent this letter hoping she would reflect on her professional practice. She had justified my section in a tribunal report. She was unclear on diagnosis and blamed me for what she called "autism traits". In some parts of the report, she lied.

I hoped that she might ask someone at rehab how they

communicate with me. God forbid, she might even ask me, or do something peculiar like involve me in my care! Or she might use Dr Mitchell to be a bridge.

Dr Malvada's office was within the autism team. She might even pop to the office next door and consult with an ASC professional. She didn't. She wrote in her notes the day I gave her the letter:

Monday 1st February, 4pm

Oxlip

Seen, angry regarding my report, difficult to engage in any any [sic] *aspect.*

Feels I do not understand her and feels threatened by me as being on section gives me the opportunity to send her to OOA (Out of Area) placement.

I said that this will be the case if her risks can not [sic] *be managed at Oxlip.*

Alexis feels she is not in control of any of that and was angry and demanding most of the interview.

Same treatment.

And this is what she wrote a week later in ward round when she hadn't read the letter.

Monday 8th February

Alexis angry as I told her that I did not have the chance to read her long letter prior to the mtg, but said I would discuss it with her there and then. Feels I do not understand her problems, said was not suicidal, all her problems are "neurological" so has not control over them. Believes the reason I don't send her to the out-of-area placement is because the team is putting pressure on me.

Wants to stay at Oxlip to be near her daughter. This past week has been good risk wise, asked two / three times to stay in.

The idea of me sending her to that placements [sic] *wakes her up at night, feels "terrified".*

I tried to engage in some positive discussions and explored what can I and the team do to make feel better. Acknowledged that waking up terrified has to be very distressing. Her daughter is going to Mexico today with her parents. Alexis showed appropriate affect when talking about it, but rapidly changed the tone and subject demanding an answer from me regarding my "formulation". Alexis said I wasn't going to cure her condition. Agreed that we could only help her to manage it.

Angry, coherent language, relevant, no evidence of thought disorder

At the end team manager put an end to the meeting as pt was getting upset and the whole conversation was running in circles.

Same treatment.

I was so upset. My fears of an OOA were right. She had confirmed them. I didn't know where to turn. This was the woman in charge of my future. Even she realised the conversations were running in circles. I was getting nowhere.

I had tried talking and now I had tried writing to her. Nothing I did could make her understand. My letter was under 1,000 words. I didn't know why she couldn't read it. Of course I was scared she would send me to an OOA placement! I wanted "treatment" at home but didn't know how to regulate myself. She could take my partial freedom away easily. In the notes she explains she will send me away if I didn't improve. I felt threatened and I felt so sad.

CHAPTER 54

Still Trying to Manage

Dr Mitchell came up with a chart. This was the only visual aid I had.

At the top was the header, 'Section 17 leave'. Underneath, a flow chart read, 'yes / no' to the following questions:

Do I feel overloaded?

Is my head full up?

To the 'yes' answers, there was a list of things I needed to do. If the answer was 'no,' then I could go out. The flow chart, as simple as it was, worked. I was very cross this hadn't been done before. I used this tool until the day I left. The danger was if I went out when I was even a little bit overloaded and it started raining, I was in trouble. Then I could easily have a meltdown and the police would come.

But when Dr Mitchell left in February, they didn't replace her. My bridge of communication was gone.

Dr Carrie told me she couldn't help me because I was too high-functioning. I asked, 'Who's going to help, then?'

She said, 'I don't know. We have to apply for funding.'

The good thing that Dr Carrie did was refer me to speech and language therapy. About two months later I was assessed by two speech and language clinicians, who agreed I needed therapy for my receptive language. They had nothing for me because I was in the mental health system. They said they might be able to send a student to help me for experience. I said, 'You're having a laugh.' Unfortunately, they weren't. Months passed and I didn't hear from them.

We sort of muddled on. I think everyone was very dejected. Dr Carrie said she would do some training with the staff, but that didn't happen either.

CHAPTER 55

Yes or No?

27th March 2016

My Mental Health Act assessment was approaching. About six weeks before the section runs out, doctors are supposed to either renew, remove, or allow it to naturally expire. Now I was in the community, involved in my child's care, and a student at university. And I was supposedly being rehabilitated from my condition.

I said to Dr Malvada six weeks before the expiration date, 'What are you going to do?'

She asked me, 'What do you think I should do?'

'Well, seeing as you're asking, I suggest you remove the section because I'm not ill, I'm not suffering from a mental health problem, and I'm not a danger.'

She said, 'You are a danger, Alexis.'

'Oh, really. How do you justify that?' I asked.

'You lack insight. You are unaware of your risks.'

'I'm not unaware. I just don't agree that I am a risk.'

Malvada replied, 'Precisely, that's the problem.'

I told her I had looked up what you need to be detained as an autistic. You must be abnormally aggressive or seriously irresponsible. I couldn't see how I was either.

She told me she would section me because I '... keep reading about death. You are fixated on it and consider it a viable option to take your life.'

I said, 'Yes, I do. But that doesn't make me a danger. Don't you get fed up with this conversation every week?'

'So, will you kill yourself?'

'Maybe, but not right now. Will you kill yourself? You probably can't answer that. Nobody can. And anyway, this is a question of ethics. You know in some countries doctors do euthanasia on people.'

She asked, 'So, what have you been reading about this week?'

'It's helium this week. It will probably be helium for a few more weeks.'

'What are you learning?'

I told her the basics of death by helium. She asked the source of my reading.

'I found a really good book online called *The Peaceful Pill*. It's research and information on informal euthanasia and assisted suicide.' When I talk about my niche interest, it's hard to hide my enthusiasm.

David had been clear about mind blindness. I was careful in these conversations to be explicit that I would not kill myself in the near future. If I ever killed myself, however, I thought I would likely use a helium method. It's easy, quick, and cheap. Importantly, it is also virtually painless. It's a popular method in many countries. I told Dr Malvada that as well.

Then she says, 'No, sorry. We can't remove the section.'

'Why not?'

'That is my decision, Alexis, and you need to accept it. We can talk again next week if you want.'

'Yes, I do want.' If Dr Malvada renewed, the section would be in place for 12 months. I couldn't face that. Also, I was stressed about having an incident and being sent to acute or even PICU. I still didn't have a handle on a lot of things.

The next week she said, 'Actually, Alexis, I've been thinking about it. I'm going to take you off the section.'

I'd had a good week. Nothing bad had happened. On hearing that, I was delighted. I told my mum and dad, my friend I had made in Oxlip – Michael, and a few of my friends. Everyone was pleased. Things were moving on. I would be a step closer to home.

Staff were not happy with the decision. They thought I would be more difficult to manage. They said the section provides boundaries which make a difference. My response was that after two weeks, I would likely go home. I didn't want to stay in hospital. I would discharge myself. I told them they needn't worry.

The following week in ward round we had the conversation again about my niche interest and also the question of whether I would remain informally. Dr Malvada had changed her mind again. This made me really cross. I could feel the emotion inside me.

'Can you just choose one or the other, please? For once give me a simple yes or no!'

'The answer, Alexis, is no. You will remain on section.'

I argued and argued. 'So, you would keep me informally if I agree to stay in hospital? Just say yes or no.'

'Yes, that is right.'

'So, I am not a danger to myself or others because I can be informal. I don't meet the criteria for detention?'

'Let's not talk about criteria. I'll worry about that. That's my job. You do need to stay in hospital so we can be sure.' Then she talked in circles. Finally, she said that the treatment would remain the same.

What treatment? I wanted to know my long-term plan. Section three was for treatment and I wasn't getting any.

Dr Mitchell had left so no psychology. There was no speech and language therapy, no sensory help, no autism-specific treatment. What was I going to be treated for 12 months for? Because if it was to learn to cook and clean, they could forget that!

There were now three weeks until my section ran out. I was getting worried and I was embarrassed. I told nobody about Malvada changing her mind, aside from my parents. I felt like this was a real power play mixed with coercion. Either I meet the criteria or I don't. Was I ill, or not? Was I a danger, or wasn't I?

I had a meeting with the unit manager, Jane, and the regional manager, Lily, on 22nd April. They assessed my risk of suicide and were satisfied I wasn't about to kill myself.

But not knowing what would happen, and Malvada's ambivalence and inability to think clearly, was stressing me out. I said, 'Look, I'm quite happy here, but I need to know. She keeps changing her mind, and it could involve a whole year for me. I want to come off the section. I'm not dangerous. I live in a house, for God's sake. I'm home three nights a week. There's no reason for me to be on section. If the risk was high, I wouldn't even be here.'

They asked about my niche interest. I told them, remembering what David had said, that it was purely an autistic special interest. Both managers seemed to understand.

They asked, 'Well, what are you going to do?'

'Of course I'm going to go home. I don't need to be in a hospital. Alright, I can't cook, but my mum can cook and go shopping. I'm not made for ADLs. I can do other things well. I have other talents.'

Both Jane and Lily were honest with me and said they were going to tell Dr Malvada I needed to remain on section. They told me they had liaised at length with the nursing team and the multidisciplinary team. They decided a renewal would be helpful as it would provide a framework to carry out a plan we created together. The plan had 14 action points. I was pleased to have a plan. I was disappointed, but I understood.

I could see a purpose and a way forward, so I was amenable. Why couldn't Dr Malvada do that? It was written on the plan that the section would be reviewed in three months. I was happy with that.

In the computerised notes, Lily wrote, 'I feel the risk is currently manageable in her current environment.'

Open doors and all, I thought.

However, on this same day Dr Malvada phoned The Priory Hospital, Hayes Grove to enquire about Keston Acute Aspergers Unit. She'd applied for a place for me in their locked unit. I didn't know until later she had done this, but I could feel she was up to something.

I spoke with my solicitor, Jessica. She would manage the section renewal, and then we would put in for a tribunal. Jessica was delighted to tell me she'd had a conversation with Dr Malvada and the good doctor had agreed to remove the section.

I said she must be mistaken. I told her about my long meeting with Jane and Lily and the 14-point plan.

Jessica was adamant this wasn't the case. She said if I agreed to stay informally and remain at the rehab, I would be discharged next week. Jessica explained that to be informal requires no specific plan. It means I could decide how long I stay.

I said I would talk to Malvada and say I would remain informally. I was looking forward to finally having a clear plan. I thanked Jessica. She knew the law so well, and I was now clear on what staying informally in rehab meant.

*

It was 25th April. During Monday ward round, I was sitting with the multidisciplinary team comprised of the nurse Sarah, Courtenay the OT, Dr Malvada, and a new junior doctor I hadn't met before.

The doctor said, 'Okay, Alexis, today we are going to remove your section. I have spoken to Jessica and we have agreed that if you will remain informally, then I will take your section off.'

'Thank you, Dr Malvada. Yes, I will stay here informally.'

'And you won't leave impulsively?'

'No, I won't.'

I could see all the staff looking at each other. I had studied facial expression in Falton Green and I knew shock when I saw it. Nurse Sarah could not hide an emotion to save her life. She was making faces and whispering to Courtenay the OT.

Dr Malvada, oblivious to what the others in the room were doing and saying, got out her pink papers. *Wow!* I thought. *She's really going to do it.* Dr Malvada asked me to sit nearer her. She showed me all the places on the pink paper she had to fill in. She asked me to shake her hand to agree that I wouldn't leave if made informal. I wasn't all that pleased to shake her hand, but I did it. She had a soft, floppy handshake.

But she didn't have a pen. She went into the office, five steps away, to get a black pen. Nurse Sarah followed her. I was left in the room with the others.

The junior doctor asked about my helium suicide plan. I hadn't met her before, so I eagerly filled her in. I said exactly what I had told the managers in a previous meeting. They had appeared to understand me, so I believed this doctor would too.

When Dr Malvada returned with the form, she said she had changed her mind after speaking to Sarah.

No member of rehab staff knew that I was to be taken off Section 3. Dr Malvada was the only person who knew, and was operating as a loose cannon!

I couldn't understand how she had changed her mind. I also couldn't understand why she hadn't filled out the paperwork the week before when she said she would. I didn't understand why she told my solicitor Jessica she would remove the section.

I didn't understand why she hadn't discussed this with managers and nursing staff before conveying such a life change to me.

All Malvada said, as if it was nothing, like she changed her mind about a drink choice at dinner, was, 'I'm sorry, Alexis, but I just spoke to Sarah, and I'm not going to remove the section.'

I felt a volcano of fire rushing into my head. Not a meltdown but a wave of righteous anger. I said to her, 'How can you show me the form, go to get the black pen, and then say you're not removing the section?' I went nuts. 'How dare you?' I said. 'Sign the form and stop playing games with me! You've been playing with me for weeks. Now just sign the fucking form!'

Then as if a spell had been cast, I couldn't speak. I couldn't locate myself in space and time. I had no idea where I was in relation to the room or people. I stumbled out the door. I went into the open office just a few steps away. I picked up a chair. I put it on my head. Not because I was going to throw it, but because the weight of it felt really nice.

The next thing I knew Nurse Sarah was putting a weighted blanket around my shoulders. Usually it helped to ground me, but it wasn't doing much today. I was just trying to pace it out. I knew if anything else happened, any more information or stimulation, I would have a meltdown.

Nurse Dawn with the ginger hair came back from shopping. I had calmed a bit. She talked to me gently. I put the chair down and spoke to her. I told her.

Dr Malvada carried on doing her ward rounds. Then the phone rang. I wasn't expecting it to ring. It pierced my ears and the shock of it was hard to manage. I picked up the phone and threw it on the floor. Telling Dawn had caused a new wave of anger. I couldn't deal with all these emotions.

I went into the ward round and started talking to Malvada. I could hardly speak. She said, 'You have to get out, Alexis. Please leave.'

I think she left the room and so did the MD team, because I stayed in the lounge. I remember Nurse Dawn with me. I was trying to get outside. Running would have helped, but Dawn wouldn't let me out. She kept standing in front of the door. I would never touch anybody, so I stayed in the room.

I put a couch over myself and stayed under there so it was pressing on me. Dawn helped. And I screamed. My head hurt so much. I was in agony.

I got around Dawn, left the rehab and ran. I ran and ran. I don't know how I got to the harbour, but I did. I am a creature of habit. I always run there. Dawn found me. I was sitting on the ground, looking at the lights. It wasn't too dark so they weren't bright.

Dawn put my blanket around me and we walked back to the rehab. I was given meds and went to bed to rest. It was a huge meltdown. Poor Dawn, she was totally knackered when she went home. I was exhausted as well, and completely out of spoons.

Staff saw my reaction as illness. I said to them, 'Look, if you took somebody's liberty away for 10 minutes for no reason, they'd be fuming. They'd be kicking the door down. If you locked them in a cage for 10 minutes, they'd go nuts. You just took my liberty away for a whole year.'

I kept that form, that pink piece of paper, my key to liberty. I still have it.

CHAPTER 56

The H5

To renew a section, the responsible clinician has to justify on an H5 form why the section is needed. To be sectioned, a person must be suffering from a mental disorder. My primary diagnosis is autism. I had secondary diagnoses of ADHD and Adjustment Disorder (Bereavement), but these did not require detention. So, to section me, Dr Malvada had to argue that my conduct, according to the Mental Health Code of Practice, must be "abnormally aggressive or seriously irresponsible".

I tried to think of why she sectioned me. I knew that I constantly displayed a compulsion to research suicide. But according to the Code of Practice 20.25, eccentricities like mine are no reason to detain on their own. Dr Malvada was aware that I was often distressed by my interest and the effect it had on people. But she did not have the specialist knowledge to assist me in disengaging from my interest and helping me to modify it. I assume this is the reason she wrote "same treatment" at the end of every ward round ... since "the same" would be more of no treatment.

In breach of the Code of Practice, Dr Malvada did not identify that the challenging behaviour I had stemmed from difficulties in communication and unmet support needs. She knew I was disturbed by even minor changes in schedule and found hospital hard. This had been recorded in my notes continuously.

I agree that I regularly demonstrated a marked difference between my intellectual and emotional development. At times this might have seemed aggressive or irresponsible. But never were specialist-structured communication approaches used for me. They might have avoided the extreme miscommunication and misunderstanding.

Dr Malvada wrote I required sectioning because I had "what Alexis refers to as a meltdown".

No, that's what it's called. I didn't make up the term. It's the name used by the autistic community and it's unique to autism. Some parents use it without knowing this when their kids have a tantrum. Like some people say that their behaviour is a little bit OCD. Dr Malvada also wrote that a meltdown is similar to a dissociative state. They can appear similar, but dissociation is caused by trauma and post-traumatic stress disorder (PTSD). A meltdown is when you can't take in any more information.

Mental health professionals regularly do not understand autism, and they also hold far too much power. If your responsible clinician doesn't understand you, then you've had it. Adult autism statutory guidance states that an MHA assessment should be conducted by an autism expert. Dr Malvada didn't bother with any specialist help.

Here is the entry from Dr Carrie:

27/04/2016 09:15:00 Dickson, Carrie

Carrie Dickson MHLD psychology Heysham

Consultation completed with Rehab and Alexis and a report written. Offer of staff support was made to Oxlip but has not been responded to. Should they require further advice I have indicated they can contact us. I will now close referral MHLD as no further need identified.

In the ward round that Monday, Dr Malvada could have sought specialist support. Her indecision every week indicated that she needed some help, especially since she was renewing a section and escalating my care.

She would have done well to call for a Care Treatment Review, a CTR, well before sectioning me. CTRs are part of the Transforming Care pathway for people with autism and / or learning disabilities. They're independent reviews to ensure services provided to autistics are appropriate. The aim is to avoid admission to hospital and escalating services by finding specialist support. It seemed Dr Malvada didn't know about this.

On 26th April 2016 she ordered another forensic assessment in the hope of getting a secure service for me. It is recorded that the precipitating event for this was my reaction to her renewal of my section for one year, after she had told me she would remove the section.

If only she had considered my communication needs when relaying the decision to me; if only she had consulted a specialist when renewing my section; if only she had ordered a CTR. Dr Malvada ignored Dr Carrie and this established pathway.

I felt like this was worse than a prison sentence. At least in prison you know when you'll be released. When you're a psychiatric patient, you're there until the responsible clinician decides you can leave. It's hard for these demi-god psychiatrists to admit that their autism-specific skills are not what they should be.

Dr Malvada used skewed information to conflate risk to justify her biased practices. Practices, I might add, that if done to the general population would be seen to infringe on human rights. I was now subject to another 12 months of control, legalised once again by the Mental Health Act.

When I complained that Dr Malvada had no clue, the trust wrote back that all doctors must complete a module on autism in medical school. I asked, 'How many years ago was that?' By the time a doctor is a consultant, it would have been a decade and half since they did that module. I did a section on learning disabilities when I was at university. I remember little except, from what I was taught, autistic people are like Rainman, Sheldon from *The Big Bang Theory* or some other media caricature.

CHAPTER 57

Unsettled

26th April to May 2016

The days after the ward round with Dr Malvada were difficult. Little things like the office door being closed most of the time added to the strained feeling between staff and me.

Dr Malvada had called in the crisis team a few hours after the ward round. HCA Lisa told me carefully about the crisis plan, using visual aids, and a written description she had printed. I was very grateful because I wasn't taking in much audibly. The plan read that the crisis team were mainly involved to support staff. They would be coming daily in pairs to promote consistency. Lisa told me they would start that evening after I had been to university.

I didn't feel like I was in a crisis. I didn't feel I needed the support. I needed people to realise that I had a normal reaction to my uncertain situation.

I photocopied a page from the *Managing Meltdowns: Using the S.C.A.R.E.D Calming Technique*[3] by Deborah Lipsky and William S. Richards. I was referred to this book in the autism ward.

It states that meltdowns will happen if:

- there is a sudden change, or being taken by surprise

- unable to understand the reasons for sudden change
- people in authority fail to explain carefully, sequentially, and descriptively what will happen next
- someone fails to respond to an autistic's questions in concrete fashion
- there is sensory overload
- asked to multitask or to integrate multiple sensory inputs

I thought this would clearly explain why I had reacted the way I did. Lisa took the paper and said she would share it with staff.

*

I went to university. It's far from rehab and I enjoyed the drive with Chester. I counted lamp posts. I was pleased to have the distraction of learning. I felt normal in the lecture hall where nobody was aware I was mental, considered in a crisis, or anything else.

I got back from university in the early evening. I told Chester I was nervous about the crisis team coming. I had to make a good impression. Chester and I discussed how I could do this and what I should say. I felt more prepared for their visit but under pressure, pressure, pressure.

As soon as I got in I asked Lisa what time the crisis team was coming. She told me they weren't coming. I could feel my brain blow up like a balloon. I started counting and pacing. Not obviously, because this would have meant I would be recorded as agitated and given meds. Lisa told me they would come the next day. It was hard enough knowing the team was involved without adding another layer of uncertainty and change.

'Will they come tomorrow?' I asked Lisa anxiously. She said they would. Of all the staff, Lisa understood. I thanked her.

*

Sitting in the TV room I had supersonic hearing. It was 26th April. Through the walls I heard that Dr Malvada had made a forensic referral. What! I couldn't believe my ears. Forensic! Me? I broke down. Those patients almost always have a history in the criminal justice system, or are perceived as such high risk that they can't be managed in a less secure facility. I don't know how Dr Malvada could make such a claim about me. I was truly helpless, hopeless, and at her mercy. And I was terrified.

Oliver from the crisis team phoned on 27th April. I asked him when he was coming. He said he wasn't coming but would phone instead. I told him I had the plan from Lisa and his phoning wasn't in it.

He ignored this and the effect it had on my anxiety. He wanted to know what was wrong and how I could get out of my "crisis". I told him I wasn't in a crisis. I explained that I was having a normal autistic reaction to unfavourable circumstances which cause overload and meltdown. He suggested that when I feel like this, I should take a bath and make a cup of tea.

'Seriously, Oliver. I need a reasonable adjustment to be made. And when they can't be made then I need strategies to manage the overload. I don't need a bath!'

And then Oliver dropped the bombshell, 'Alexis, you will get that at the autism out-of-area placement you're going to.'

'The what? What are you talking about?'

'You know, out-of-area, OOA, placement for autism.'

'Yah, I know what an OOA is. But I'm not going anywhere.'

'You are going where we tell you, Alexis. You should be pleased. It's in London and costs a lot of money. A bed will be available soon.'

I dropped the phone and cried and cried. I said to Dawn, 'What about my daughter? I won't see her. How will I take her to school and pick her up? And my running club? When will I get to run with them? I have marathons booked next month. I go home three nights a week! I can't go to London. I have to go home three times ... I must go home and see my daughter and my friends. When will I see them? I'm part of a community, you know. I have to go to university. I can't get here from London. I'm in the middle of a course. And that OOA is a locked ward. I need the door open. I like the garden and the feeling of freedom ... and ... and ...'

I was assured by ward staff that no decision had been made. It was speculative. Dawn and Lisa told me they knew nothing of it. 'Perhaps it was being discussed but it isn't a sure thing.' This settled me a lot. Back in 2013 and 2014, I had been told many things that didn't happen. Nothing was certain.

But the following day, I was in constant overload. When overloaded, I can't go out on my own, so I asked Lily, the service manager, for help. Lily had been a runner in the past. The previous week, I'd run a marathon and she had given me tips. She knew how important running was for me.

Lily drove me to the coastal cliff so I could run for 36 minutes. My pace was way faster than usual. I enjoyed the feeling of my feet hitting the ground. The feedback through my body felt great.

Lily waited in the car for me, working on her laptop. After my 6k run, I apologised for being sweaty. She said she didn't mind. 'Do you feel better?' she asked.

'Yes,' I said.

I came back to rehab and was waiting to cook dinner with Dawn. She was going to help me make a dish and we would eat together. Oliver from the crisis team phoned again just as we were about to start. I asked him why they weren't coming in pairs as it says in my written plan. Oliver said it was because I was doing okay. He apologised for telling me the news about the OOA.

'It's okay, Oliver,' I said. 'At least nothing is decided. I might even stay here. No harm done.'

'Er, Alexis, you are going to the autism unit. You need to know that. You are going for at least three months. It'll be a trial period to assess you.'

My brain went **ROOOOOOM** – the worst thing that could possibly happen. Not just because a meltdown is horrible but because it would affect my future.

I ran from the house. I was stopped by the police. A member of rehab saw me at the harbour and drove back to tell Dawn, who came and got me. I was lifted into the police van and Dawn sat next to me. That's commitment. She could have just left me to get handcuffed and caged. In fact, she could have just not bothered with me. The police stayed with Dawn for a while in rehab to make sure I didn't leave. Dawn worked for two hours to bring me closer to functional. I didn't know any of what had happened. I was informed by another nurse, who enjoyed telling me what an inconvenience I was.

I was exhausted when I went to bed that night. Totally out of spoons, I couldn't speak or coordinate my steps well to get up the stairs. I made a cup of tea, which was an effort, and I spilt hot water. I tried to relax but my mind wouldn't switch off.

All was not as it seemed. I wasn't sure if I could trust Oxlip staff. Were they lying to me? Would an ambulance come and get me in the middle of the night? I didn't know who to trust, and once again I didn't feel I was being included in my future.

It was 27th April. I had two settled days after that. No crisis team. Things were rather odd with staff. I heard mentions of PICUs and medium secure facilities, which I ignored.

CHAPTER 58

The Cliff

On 30th April, I woke up tearful as I had done since the section was renewed. In overload, my brain just wouldn't switch off. I was still trying to work out why things were so bad. Unable to settle, I asked Nurse Ethel to take me for a run on the cliffs. We drove in silence. As usual, my named nurse Ethel knew just what to say and do.

It was a bright, sunny day and Ethel rolled down the windows on her little car. The warm breeze entered and blew "feedback" into my face. I was again oriented to space and time.

We got out of the car and walked the short distance to the promenade. The sea was a beautiful blue and waves were gently crashing on the beach. It was curious to watch the water disappear through the pebbles as if it had never been there. I thought of my own situation where psychiatry, like the water, felt insurmountable but then magically would disappear without a trace.

We walked to a bench where I assumed Nurse Ethel would sit and wait. I turned to her. 'I'm wearing my pyjamas! For goodness' sake! What is wrong with me?'

'I thought you knew that, Alexis.'

'Of course I didn't. When do I ever run in my pyjamas?'

'Some patients are too exhausted to get changed when they're depressed. You looked tired so I didn't mention it.'

'Yeah, I am tired. But I can't run like this.'

'No problem, Lexi. Let's sit here and just chat. It's a beautiful day.'

After an hour of discussing what might happen, Nurse Ethel said it was time to go. I was really enjoying the sun and the quiet sound of the waves and asked her if I could stay. She reluctantly agreed.

I walked along the promenade and found a nice piece of cliff. I hopped over the waist-high fence and sat on a one-metre ledge watching the water. The cliff was sloping, but steeper than the type I used to roll down as a child.

I calculated the drop. It's a habit. You know, it's not the height of the fall that kills you, it's the sudden stop at the bottom. The most detailed data on the effects of large accelerations, or actually decelerations, on the human body comes from research into spaceflight and aircraft ejection systems.

I sat there thinking how shit my life was. I was upset and tearful.

A young boy rode up on his bike and set it down on the bench behind me. He sat too, looking out over the sea. I noticed him because I thought it unusual for a boy in his late teens to be doing this. When I looked at him again, he said, 'Hello.'

I said, 'Hi.'

'Nice day, eh,' he said. Here comes the small talk. *I asked for this*, I thought to myself. I asked his name – Meshack.

'You look upset. Are you okay?' he asked.

Is it that obvious? I guess I must have looked odd in my PJs. And I had big black eyes from lack of sleep. I told him I was sad.

We started chatting. He told me his dad had just died. I felt very upset and said, 'Oh, that's awful.'

He sat next to me but behind me. We talked for a long time. Meshack got a little emotional too. He was a nice boy and asked a lot about my life. I don't know what he thought, except in that moment we shared a conversation about loss. I was unaware I was attracting attention.

A person passing asked, 'Are you alright?'

I said, 'I'm fine,' and kept looking at the water.

Then it happened again. I said, 'I'm just chatting with this boy.'

And again. We were talking for ages before I was aware there were groups of people looking at us.

I asked Meshack about it. He said they were just worried about me. I panicked after another person asked, 'Are you okay? Can you come back over the railing?'

I knew I was overloaded and talking more slowly. It took a while to respond. I said, 'No, I'm just looking at the sea. There's nothing wrong with that.'

Someone said, 'I think you need to come back over, love.'

I kept saying, 'No, thank you.' Then I realised. *Shit. They think I'm going to jump off.*

There was now a crowd of people behind me.

The reality of what was happening dawned on me. I was on a section. I was detained in a place where the doctor doesn't want me. She was trying to move me to a locked unit. The doctor was inflating risk and I'd just helped her do this because I was sitting on a cliff and people were thinking I wanted to jump. *I'm not getting out of this.*

My head was totally full as all this flooded my mind.

I could just go back over the railing. But if I did that, would they transfer me to locked? I was in total panic.

Meshack and I had gone from having a meaningful conversation to him panicking and wondering what to do with me. How on earth had this happened?

Although ever the logical one, I could find no good way out. It was like being back in Falton Green, on the same day a year ago, looking at that beautiful blue sky and wanting to "go to sleep". Believe me, the irony was not lost on me. I felt trapped again. For a fleeting moment, I considered jumping.

A police officer came. I hate when they try to help me. Their interventions never end well. This small female officer started chatting to me. But her talk was hurting my ears. She was trying to persuade me to come back over. I told her I wasn't stupid, and I knew that she would arrest me as soon as I did. I told her that I felt stuck and I wasn't sure what do next. Until I had thought everything through, I wouldn't be moving.

The officer asked if I was going to jump. I told her it was unlikely. Despite the apparent hopelessness of my situation, I wasn't 100% sure. I told her to leave but she wouldn't. I tried to reassure her, 'Data suggests that to be sure of death you have to travel at more than 12 metres per second impact velocity. Anything less and you're almost certain to survive. This corresponds to a fall from a height of just over 7 metres, which I don't have here. The result would be survival with life-changing injuries. No thanks. So, no, officer, I won't jump.'

She said, 'Come back over and we can sort it all out.'

Then Nurse Ethel came. She asked, 'Can you come back over now, Lexi?'

Oh, my goodness. PLEASE give me some space to think. I don't know what to do. None of you have my best interests at heart. Let me think.

After some time refusing to come back over the fence, I managed to say, 'Ethel, I'm only coming back if you promise me we can go to rehab.'

'Yeah, I promise, Lexi.'

'Seriously?' I saw nobody else except her and the police officer and a few people looking.

She said, 'Look, there's my car.'

I said, 'Go and get your car.'

She said again – I made her say it – 'I promise we're going straight to Oxlip.' So, she went to get her car.

This whole thing had taken probably 45 minutes. That was around the usual time for me to recover. So, I climbed over the fence, said goodbye to Meshack, and got into Ethel's car. I had just shut the door when about 15 police officers appeared from behind bushes, dustbins, and seemingly out of thin air. They ran at us.

I screamed at Nurse Ethel, 'You fucking liar. You lied to me.'

She said, 'I didn't lie.' She was crying and screaming.

The officers grabbed me out of the car, smashed me onto the ground, and handcuffed me. I was no longer in a meltdown. I was shouting at them, 'Can you fucking get off me, you bastards?' Nurse Ethel was howling with fright.

I yelled at her, 'Will you shut up?' I was on the ground with my hands handcuffed behind my back. My legs were being tied together. 10 to 15 officers all piled on top of me and around me.

I kept saying, 'Get off me, get off me.'

An inspector came over and calmed Ethel down.

I asked them again, 'Can you get off me, you bastards?'

They said, 'Okay, but are you going to be alright, Alexis? You're not going to run or kick out at us?'

'How can I run all tied up like this?' I said. 'I've never hurt anybody.' So, they untied my legs and let me stand up, my hands still handcuffed behind my back, two officers holding me. Fire burnt beneath my arms where they were holding me, and my clothes scratched my skin.

I asked them again to let go. 'That feels like fire, so can you get off my arms?'

They said, 'Not yet.' They phoned the crisis team. Apparently, I put myself in a high-risk situation. I tried arguing that the ledge was a metre wide and I wouldn't fall, but to no avail. I pointed to a person sitting on the other side of the fence, but no one was interested in that.

'Look!' I said, pointing to the cliff. 'I was fully aware of the risks, having calculated the height and rate of acceleration and deceleration on impact. I wasn't being risky or careless. I wouldn't have died.' They were being irrational, not me.

Eventually they took off the handcuffs and said, 'We're sorry we had to do that, Alexis.' They all knew me. 'Just go back to Oxlip with Nurse Ethel. The crisis team has decided you return to Oxlip. We are not happy about that, but there are no beds in the acute units for you.'

I talked to Ethel on the way back. I was very confused about why people had reacted the way they did and how things had escalated so quickly. I concluded it was another case of mind blindness where I didn't realise what other people were thinking until it was too late. Ethel also insisted my actions were dangerous and that I lacked insight into risky behaviour. I told her I had done much riskier things overseas that including scaling waterfalls.

That evening I replayed in my head the police coming at me and throwing me to the ground. I didn't sleep well.

*

The following day, Nurse Sarah was on shift. As usual, she talked about how risky my behaviour had been. I assured her that in no way was I at risk. But again, I was told I lacked insight. 'Sarah, I see loads of people sitting in that same spot watching the waves all the time. It isn't dangerous. People sit there.'

'They are not on a section, Lexi.'

'Nope, I guess they aren't.'

She didn't let me go out on my own that day. I went for a walk with Lisa to get my shopping. It was bright and noisy inside, but I managed. I baked a cake in the afternoon.

CHAPTER 59

Now What?

May 2016

Things seemed to go back to normal until Thursday 5th May. I went for a run every day for between 30 minutes and a couple of hours. I took Abi to and from school, to play with her friends, and I went out for hot chocolate. On a rare occasion I went shopping with my mum to the mall.

I was unaware that behind the scenes Dr Malvada had made the referral to move me to a more secure unit. She tried acute, but they wouldn't take me because in the commissioner's eyes what was the difference between acute and rehab? Then she made a referral to Ivy Suite PICU. They refused to accept me because of my diagnosis. Based on this, she made a referral to the private London PICU, Slade at Beckton. That awful place had no beds. Ivy didn't want me to have to go in an OOA PICU, so they agreed to an assessment to take me back.

I was reminded again that there was no place for high-functioning autistic women in the system.

On Thursday, I was going about my business. I noticed Nurse Ethel's name had been replaced on the staffing board. More than the discomfort this caused me, I felt sorry if it was because of me.

As I went to the TV room, I saw Shyam. I thought I was seeing things. He looked at me and then walked into the staff office. The door closed. I wasn't seeing things. I didn't think more of it. Everything was going well.

Later, Shyam re-emerged. I said, 'Hi, Shyam! How are you doing?' I gestured to shake his hand and we hugged instead. 'It's so great to see you.'

He said, 'I'm annoyed, Lexi, that I have to be here.'

'Why?'

'Because I have to discuss you again.' He said it in an almost sad way, like *You were doing so well, why am I here?*

'I don't know why you're here, Shyam.' Then it dawned on me ... 'Yeah, why is he here?' I asked, to no one, insistent for a reply.

He said, 'I'll come and speak to you in a bit.' He was PICU Outreach which was the gatekeeping service for Ivy Suite. The Outreach service decided whether you met the criteria for admittance. Dr Malvada had referred me because she believed I was trying to commit suicide. She had escalated my risk again. But she knew I was well versed in suicide and if I had wanted to die, I would already be dead!

Shyam was in the office for a long time. Then he came and found me in the TV lounge and asked, 'What's all this stuff I'm hearing about you? That you are suicidal and aggressive.'

'I'm not, Shyam. That's a lie.'

He heard me and said, 'This is the best I've ever seen you. I have never been called to see somebody who needs a PICU less than you. But Lexi, you've got to stop this behaviour.'

'I know. I wish I could. I don't know how. I hate myself. Especially at times like this. But I'll try harder. I'm going to try harder.' I was begging him, desperate.

'How?'

'Right now, I don't know, but I'm going to look it up on the internet.'

'Good, Lexi. You must. Dr Malvada wants to move you to a more secure facility.'

He had to come again the next day for another assessment. He said, 'Lexi, they're trying to send you to the London PICU. You know you've been referred for forensic, right?'

'No, no, no, she can't. That place traumatised me. I'll never get out of there. You know here, I get overloaded like once a fortnight. In there it was every couple of hours. I can't do that again. And it's actually dangerous in there. I'm scared, Shyam. Please don't let them send me,' I begged him.

'The doctor wants you out of here. You have to stay calm. Remember what Achala and I always told you, "It's in your hands."'

I remembered that I had told Achala that it was going to be the last time I'd see her on my last admission, that I wasn't going to be readmitted to Ivy.

Except it clearly wasn't.

Shyam left and I went to the gym and for a run. At least my routine was the same. That kept me sane. I was coping.

On Friday, Shyam came. 'You are not going to London PICU. You would have had to go there if we didn't accept you. Lexi, we had refused to take you. That's why you were referred. But Dr Saty (the Ivy Suite RC) and I have discussed it and we will take you at Ivy. We know how to manage you.'

'Why, Shyam? Why do I have to go to a PICU?'

'First, you don't meet the criteria for PICU. That's why we refused you. You are doing fine here in an open community unit. We also refused you because you are autistic and Ivy cannot manage autism. It is not an appropriate environment. That's why Dr Malvada tried to send you to the London PICU, to circumvent Ivy Suite's decision that you're not suitable for PICU. The Slade at Beckton said they would accept you, but they had no beds.'

'But Slade PICU is even less appropriate,' I argued.

'Anyway, Lexi, we have been told to do a 72-hour assessment with a view to taking you on Monday.'

'But nothing's happened, Shyam. The last five days have been fine. I don't need to be locked up.' I said this knowing it would make absolutely no difference. I said it knowing my life was about to be turned upside down. I was about to re-enter the system, where I would react badly to the environment and be made insane.

That day Dr Malvada called me into her office and removed all of my Section 17 leave five days after the cliff incident. Why? I didn't know.

I was now confined to Oxlip. I couldn't leave the back garden. I couldn't pick my daughter up, go running, go to the gym, go to university. I couldn't go shopping for my own food.

Dr Malvada had exerted her power again. And for what? Was this supposed to help me? If I wanted to escape, I could just walk out of the front door. What was the point of removing my leave? It was a punishment. To show she had the power, maybe?

I didn't know.

*

I spent most of my time in the garden. I knew soon I could find myself in a medium secure unit surrounded by a five-metre fence. So, I sat on the waist-high gate with my legs dangling, trying to take in what was about to happen. All my hope was gone.

I could do nothing to help myself now. I hadn't explored other ways to manage. Over these eight months, Oxlip had taken me as an institutionalised person and taught me everything I needed to do in the community. I had become semi-independent.

Talk about a return to poor self-concept! Now I was labelled as uncooperative, belligerent, disruptive, and out of control.

What would become of me? I had no way to use my coping strategies. Dr Malvada had no alternative plan in place to help. This put me at high risk of sensory overload and meltdown. With no means to cope, I was regressing to how I had been in acute. I started stimming badly. I knew these movements were coming back to help me manage, but they were distressing.

Shyam came to see me on Saturday as he had told me. I said, 'I want my fucking leave back. I want to go to university on Wednesday to complete my course work and I really need to run.'

'She won't give it back at the moment, Lex.'

'Can you ask Dr Saty to give it back?'

Shyam said, 'He's not your responsible clinician. Look, this is what we will do. I'm going to assess you today. On Sunday, Mishan will come. You remember him, the Ivy ward manager?'

I asked, 'Why isn't a bog-standard PICU Nurse coming to assess me? Why are you sending the deputy ward manager and the ward manager?'

'Lexi, this is serious. Big decisions are being made and people can't agree. On Monday we've got a meeting with the directors of Kingshire and Heysham NHS Trust to decide what to do with you. But don't worry. If you go anywhere, I'm taking you to Ivy Suite.'

'Do I have a say in this, Shyam?'

'You know that's not how things are done, Lexi.'

'I don't want to go to Ivy Suite! I don't need to go there. And from Ivy Suite, where am I going? I'll kick off there. Now I only have a meltdown every few weeks, not every few hours. I can't live like this, Shyam. I'm going to university, mate. I'm in the middle of a course. I have a running club. I'm a member of this community now. I live at home three nights a week. After school, Abi asks, 'Are you coming home, mummy?' And I have to say, 'No, sweetheart, I have to work.' I tell her I'm at work because she's only four years old. You can't do this, Shyam. You can't put me in a cage. I'm not going in a cage, and I'm not living in Ivy Suite. Where would I go from there?'

He said, 'We've identified this locked unit – Keston. It's part of the Priory.'

'I'm not going to Keston. And I'm not going to any medium security either. I have a life here.'

'Well, they think what you did on the cliff was really dangerous. You'll go where you are taken.'

'It wasn't dangerous,' I said. 'People sit and look out at the water. I'm sick and tired of you people telling me I'm dangerous. I'm not dangerous.'

'You lack insight and that's not your fault.'

'Do you really believe that? I can't believe the directors are involved.'

'Well, you're such a high-risk case, Lexi, it's had to go all the way up to the directors.'

'I'm not high risk. Do you really think I'd be in a rehab if I was that bad?'

'I know, but just because of your history.'

'You created that history.' I had researched Keston and it was for autistics with learning disabilities. 'I've been to one of those already, and I'm certainly not going back. The last time I came to you, I came from Falton Green, the money-making hospital. I don't want to go to another private hospital. I don't want to go to hospital, actually. Can you just take the stupid section off?'

*

On Sunday, when the Ward Manager Mishan came, I was really strong. I said, 'Let's not pretend this is about risk. It's about Dr Malvada who doesn't want me in her unit. She sectioned me so she could force me away. And she is inflating perceived risk.'

'Really, Lexi, you don't think she has a point?'

'No, I don't! She has taken my leave to force me into a crisis. On the 30th April, at the cliff, my coping strategies didn't work. Why? I was really tired. I have been under a lot of stress caused mostly by Dr Malvada. I had been sectioned for a year for no reason, gotten upset when Dr Malvada teased me with the section form, plus I was referred to forensic services. Therefore, Mishan, when you assess my risk today and back at the cliff, know that the adverse effects of my autism are sizeable. The extent to which these stressors, my faulty theory of mind, and language issues had an impact is huge. This must be clear when comparing my usual functioning to my impairments. Tell that to the directors! And tell them these should not have occurred, and it's unfair to punish me.'

Mishan said, 'Well, nothing is definite yet. Let's see on Monday. Ideally you can stay here until a bed is available in Keston. But that will take three to six months, I think. If worse comes to worse, you will come to Ivy with us and you will wait for the bed there.'

'I'm not coming with you. Please don't do this, Mishan.'

'Well, we'll see what the directors say.'

I went to bed Sunday night thinking that my life was over. I had two choices here. I could die. I could easily kill myself. If I was going to kill myself, I had to do it now because I was in a house. As soon as I got to Ivy Suite, it wouldn't be possible. I would go to Ivy and await transfer to Keston. I could never come back through the NHS pathway, which is Ivy Suite, acute unit, rehab.

CHAPTER 60

New Plan

9th May 2016

I needed a plan. I had to move fast. Going to a locked unit wasn't an option. I considered death and quickly ruled that out. I wasn't about to let Malvada kill me.

If I stayed in rehab even a few more hours I could have been transferred. Perhaps death was the only way out. But I realised it couldn't be.

I went from hopelessness to hope. Oxlip had rehabilitated me. I had skills and I could make it. I was functional. I was fine. I wasn't sick. I was just autistic, and I didn't want to die.

I had to leave.

By now, I was very familiar with mental health law. The Mental Health Act is only valid in England and Wales. Scotland has an agreement to transfer any AWOL or OOA patients back to England, so Scotland was out of the question. Also, it would have taken too long to get to there.

But rehab wasn't far from Dover. Dover is in southeast England and is home to the Channel Tunnel, the fastest way to France where I would be out of range of the MHA.

Okay, I needed to get to Dover. But you had to check in for the tunnel like in an airport. They could track that. What else could I do? I could take the ferry. You can buy tickets and just walk straight on. That seemed the most logical solution. When I got to France, I'd be free.

Upon realising this as the best and quickest solution, I thought a little further. It was too expensive in France. What little money I had wasn't going to be enough.

The solution: a developing country. This made sense because I could live for at least two months to get the section off. Then I'd return. It wasn't a long-term solution, but it would give me time to come up with a better plan for the rest of my life.

I remembered that my friend Jaz had just moved to West Africa. I messaged Jaz on Facebook and said, 'Do you fancy a visitor?' She knew nothing about what had been happening. The whole time this had been happening, I'd been keeping up a façade on Facebook of my lovely life with Abi as best I could.

She said, 'Yeah, that would be amazing. Come over. I can't wait to see you. When are you thinking of coming?'

'Within the next two days, mate. I'll let you know.' Jaz was a bit shocked to hear that it was so soon, but I hadn't seen her for years and she said she was looking forward to catching up.

By this time, much of the night had passed. My plan was in place logistically. Now to iron out the finer details.

Where was the nearest international airport to Calais? I looked at flights from Charles de Gaulle in Paris to West Africa. But I didn't want to fly direct. I don't know why. It just didn't sit well with me.

I looked at ferry times, found a train from Calais to Paris and earmarked a flight via Dubai.

When it was five o'clock in the morning, I phoned home. Having no intention of talking to my law-abiding, ex-police officer mother, I was pleased when Dad answered.

'Dad, I need my passport.'

He said, 'For what?'

'I'm going to Africa. I'm going today.'

'You don't need to persuade me, Lex. Have you organised yourself?'

'Yes, pretty much,' I said.

'Good. I'll bring it when I drop Abi off at school,' he said. 'The only thing is, I don't think your mum is going to allow this. How are you getting to Calais?'

'I don't know yet.'

'Do you want me to drive you?'

'No, you can't. It's illegal. They'll come for Abi. They'll take her, saying you and Mum are irresponsible.'

This was the last piece of the plan I hadn't sorted out. Who on earth could I ask to do such a thing? To break the law? Who believed in me? Few people now, I was sad to admit.

I phoned Jenny and David. They were the only ones I knew that believed in me enough and were sufficiently disillusioned with the system to do something this crazy. It was early morning, about seven o'clock when Jenny answered. I wasn't sure what to say. There aren't scripts you can learn for this type of request. So, I got straight to the point.

'Jenny, you know you keep saying you want to kidnap me? Can you kidnap me today?'

Jenny and David fully knew the gravity of the situation. Jenny wanted to hear my plan in detail. David and she were not people to do something without ensuring it would work out.

After I had explained everything, Jenny said, 'Right. We'll be there.'

'I have to leave before one o'clock because that's when the directors' meeting is. We must go this morning.'

'The earliest I can get there is ten o'clock. I'll wake David and drive straight away.'

Meanwhile, news had travelled to my mum. My dad didn't let her talk to me on the phone because she was hysterical.

I could hear her in the background, 'You can't do this. You can't do this. This is the wrong way to do it.'

Dad told her, 'There isn't a right way. We tried. We've given them three-and-a-half years. There's no other way.' Mum just kept crying. We didn't include her in the plan because she wasn't able to be included. She knew nothing of what was happening apart from the fact that I was about to escape the country.

Mum took her own action and phoned Jenny up. Jenny said, 'Look, I'm doing it, and I hope one day you'll forgive me. She must be rescued. They're going to lock her up for years. I'm not having a person of sound mind and who has committed no crime being incarcerated. I am doing the right thing. This is a humanitarian issue.'

Mum told her we could fight it.

'You can't fight these people. You can't fight huge institutions with all of their power, money, and invested interest.'

Over the next hour, I did my best to stay as insanely "normal" as possible. I ate breakfast. I did my chores. I dutifully went for my meds. I'm not good at lying so when they asked me how I was, I said I was nervous. When they asked what I would do that day, I said I would spend the day outside.

My dad arrived at 8.45am with Abi. I played football with her in the garden for 15 minutes, because she started school at nine o'clock. It was a lovely, sunny day. I didn't want to raise any alarms, so my dad brought nothing with him except a brown envelope which he handed me. I checked when I was upstairs. Inside was my passport, £100, and €30.

Just before nine o'clock, Dad and Abi left. This was hard. Really hard. I was about to be free. I was entering the unknown. I hugged him. Then I hugged Abi for a super-long time.

She said, 'I'll see you after school today, Mummy. We can play football.'

'Yes, darling, I'll see you after school. I love you.'

'I love you too, Mummy.'

That was the last time I saw her for months.

I went upstairs. I couldn't stop thinking about how this was all real, that it was happening.

I questioned whether I was doing the right thing for Abi. I realised if I went to Keston in London or Ivy Suite there would be no phone, no internet. I wouldn't see her. I didn't want to miss any more of her life. I rationalised that by getting back my life I would also give her the relationship with me she deserved.

I phoned Jenny to let her know everything was going to plan. I had the passport and had packed my backpack. Over the next hour, I had to act normally. This wasn't very difficult because I like the routine.

At 9.30am, I took part in the morning meeting. Since it was Monday, the nurse allocated our chores. It was the bloody kitchen for me, so I spent my last morning cleaning the kitchen.

Then I got my backpack from upstairs and put it in the garden behind the wheelie bins. Inside the backpack were two sets of underwear, running trousers, three shorts, and three T-shirts. I added two books and my passport. That was all I had space for.

After the bag had been safely stowed out of sight, I played outside in the garden. I sat periodically on the waist-high brick fence thinking how ridiculous the situation was. My phone was in my pocket. I had set it to vibrate.

David and Jenny called when they were five minutes away. They pulled up and I quickly jumped into the car. David drove at a sensible speed to Dover and arrived in good time. Nobody followed us. I felt oddly out of place as a mental patient in a public arena.

I bought a ticket for David, Jenny, me, and their car. I should have bought me a ticket as a foot passenger, and David and

Jenny as the car, to separate us but this didn't occur to me or them until much later.

No person may assist a detained patient in actions against their section. I had no Section 17 leave, so when I left that building they were breaking the law. Here is the section which describes the criminal offence:

Section 128 – **the offence of assisting someone to go AWOL or of harbouring them whilst AWOL:** this would cover helping someone to leave hospital when they are detained under the MHA and it would include allowing them to stay with you or supplying with assistance of various kinds, if you know they are AWOL under the Act.[4]

We went through the usual checks on the English side of the channel. So far, so good. I distracted myself by counting. David and Jenny were very calm, which helped.

We got on the ferry and found seats upstairs. I wasn't at all hungry, but David and Jenny hadn't eaten so they ordered coffee and pastries. I was gently rocking in my place and David drew my attention to it. He reminded me that I was now free.

It was a sunny day, so after they finished their breakfast we went out on the deck. I looked down at my arm and saw my wristband, "Medical Alert" with my name, diagnosis, and Oxlip telephone number. I tossed it into the sea between England and France. This was the most liberating feeling I'd ever had. I glanced up at the white cliffs of Dover in the beautiful sunlight. I was so emotional.

Overhead, I could see two helicopters flying along the coast. Jenny joked that they were looking for me. It turns out they were looking for me, but I would find that out later. Police cars were also patrolling the area. I didn't text my dad because I was afraid the police might check his phone.

The ferry landed in the Calais harbour. Jenny and David said, 'Right. This is the moment of truth.' Freedom was nearly mine.

David pulled the car out of the ship. As we drove along French soil towards the French gendarme, the border patrol waved us through. They didn't even look at my passport. I cried tears of relief. Tears of freedom.

Jenny and David were planning to drop me at the train station in Calais, but they decided they would drive me to Charles de Gaulle. It was a two-hour drive. I was so grateful. After that I would be on my own.

Jenny got a message from my dad saying the police had been at our family home all morning, searching the house. They even searched the attic. My mother was still in floods of tears. She was asking them, 'How can you possibly have lost my daughter?'

My dad had said, 'Maybe she is on a long run.' How right he was! A long run indeed.

In central Paris, David and Jenny dropped me at the airport. I hopped out with my backpack, and they drove off. Jenny said, 'Just text me when you get through immigration.'

I went to Emirates Airlines and bought a ticket for Lagos. Emirates stops in Dubai.

I love airports. Because of their order, I don't find them overloading. I like the A, B, C designations, and each letter's allocation of desks. Everything is so organised. I know the Dubai airport well. I used it as a main hub when I lived in Asia. I felt comfortable knowing I would land there.

Everything was fine so far. No problem buying the ticket. I got through security and was in the line for immigration. So far, so good.

I stood patiently at the yellow line waiting my turn. The immigration officer called me forwards. I handed him my passport and ticket. He scanned my passport and waved me through. Phew.

I had just stepped past the booth when he called out, 'Excuse me. Come back,' in a thick French accent.

I asked him, 'What's the problem, mate?'

He said, 'I don't speak English.'

I said, 'Well, you do. What's the problem?' In less than a minute, four armed police were standing around me. I stood behind his desk for what seemed like ages. I wasn't worried at this stage because I had committed no crime.

The French police uniforms are different from British uniforms. I didn't have the same stress reaction. I was fine. So, I got on the phone and called Jenny. She asked, 'Do you want me to come back?'

'You can't come back,' I said.

'No, no, I'll come back,' Jenny replied and we had a mini-debate. 'They need to know your condition.'

'No, they don't. It's irrelevant. I'm okay. I'm not going to melt down. Anyway, you'll be arrested if you come back.' The magnitude of what they had done for me was great. I hoped in that moment and for the next six months they would be okay. A criminal conviction for the crime they committed would have seriously affected them.

Jenny said, 'We've just heard from your dad. The British police are still with them.'

I spoke to the French police in French, 'What's the problem?'

They said again, 'We don't speak English.'

I thought, *Yes, you do speak English.* I kept my cool and waited. I said, 'I have my ticket. Just let me get on the plane. I'll leave France. I will not cause you any problem.'

They kept saying, 'I don't understand you, I don't speak English.'

After about 30 minutes, I embarked on what I can only describe as a scene out of Border Control. Marched along winding corridors underneath Charles de Gaulle airport, I was petrified not knowing where I was going. With only a substandard TV show for reference, I was worried that I was going to be locked in a psychiatric hospital in bloody France. We went into a bland room where there were four or five computers and loads of French police.

The police at their desks paid little attention to me. There was nowhere to run and what good would running do anyway? I kept reminding myself I hadn't done anything wrong. I sat down. That didn't last long. So, I paced the 15-metre stretch of space between me and the police. Once again, I became oriented to my space.

Finally, I said to an officer who was sitting at a desk, 'Look, mate. What's the problem here?'

He said, 'I don't speak English.'

I said, 'Let me just talk at you, and see if you understand anything. You've detained me. I can see you don't know why. I don't speak much French, but I have gathered that. I am going to tell you why you've detained me. Do you understand me so far?'

'Yes,' said the officer. He had turned towards me now and was listening. I had his full attention.

'It's because I'm an escaped psychiatric patient. This morning I fled England from a psychiatric rehabilitation unit. I have autism. The doctor was planning on sending me to a secure unit. I didn't agree with her and so I fled the country.'

'Oh, is that what it is?'

I thought, *So, he speaks English now.*

He says, 'How did you escape?'

'That's not really any of your concern, but I have escaped. I'm on my way to Dubai. Look, you can clearly see I'm not mentally ill. I mean, what patient suffering from severe mental illness can do what I have just done?'

'Yes. That is a good point. But you see the English Home Office have put a marker on your passport. We are obliged to stop you.'

'The British police are with my father now. But they have no jurisdiction here according to my research on the Mental Health Act. And you can see I am well.'

I spent 10 minutes trying to convince him I was fine. I showed him photos on my phone. Thankfully, they were all dated. He could see that two weeks ago I had done a marathon. I had a picture of me running and my medal after. I showed him pics of me at university in the coffee lounge. My iPhone has the GPS facility that shows where you are, so he could see that too. I showed the officer me running with my running club friends and finally I showed him my daughter. By this time three police were all looking at my phone.

'You can see, guys, I'm not mental. I just don't want to be in a psychiatric hospital. I'm a teacher. There's nothing wrong with me. Anyway, you've got no legal jurisdiction over me here. The Mental Health Act does not apply in France, and I've not committed a crime.'

He said, 'Oh, my God, I can't believe you've escaped from a psychiatric hospital. What idiots to have had such lax security. If you are that crazy, how did you end up here?'

'Yeah, well, I don't agree with everything you just said. However, I have escaped, and you can see there's nothing wrong.'

He said, 'Yeah, okay. Let me talk to the British police.' So, I phoned my dad and he gave the phone to the police. I spoke to them first.

They asked, 'Where are you, Alexis?'

I said, 'I'm in Paris.'

'You're in Paris?' There was a stunned silence. 'Paris? In France?'

'Yeah, I'm with the French police. They've detained me, you bastards. You want to take the red flag off my fucking passport, because you have no jurisdiction over me here?'

The French policeman gestured for the phone. In very good English, he chatted with the English police.

After the call, the French policeman told me, 'If they don't call back within an hour and a half, you can catch your flight.'

'Right, okay.' I phoned Dad back.

'The French police have given the English police a deadline. But if the English police can find something in the Mental Health Act that says they can continue to detain me, I'll be deported back to England.'

My parents' house suddenly became a research centre into the MHA. Apparently, the English police were all sitting around our dining-room table googling Mental Health Act, absconding, AWOL, etc. But they couldn't find anything.

I called Jessica, my solicitor, but couldn't reach her.

Dad told me the English police tried to get the Mental Health Act office to assist, but they came up with nothing. Did I expect anything else? Nope.

He said, 'I just keep showing them where it says jurisdiction England and Wales only.'

I said, 'Just keep doing that.'

In the meantime, I had connected with the French police guy. I wished all my communication was this easy. We were chatting away. We talked about Brexit. He said, 'We French want a Frexit. We are sick of Europe.' We talked about all the immigration problems they have at the airport and in Calais.

When the hour and a half passed, he said, 'Right. Time's up. Let's go.'

I cried a bit. I hadn't felt so much emotion for a long time. I phoned Dad and said, 'I'm going, Dad. I'm going.'

Dad said, 'Yeah!' I could hear my mum crying and howling in the background. I spoke to Abi.

She said, 'I'll come and see you tomorrow, Mummy.'

'You'll see me soon, baby girl, I can promise you that,' I replied, choking back tears. Nobody should have to do what I was doing.

CHAPTER 61

Free

The only good thing about being held up for so long was that I was escorted by the French policeman from the detention area straight to the plane.

I found my seat. I was so relieved. I'll never forget my feeling of liberation as I waited to take off. While we were on the runway, I phoned Oxlip.

I said, 'Hi!'

They said, 'Is that you, Alexis? Where are you? You must come back.'

I said, 'Have the police not spoken to you?'

They said, 'No. Where are you?'

'I'm on an airplane now.'

'What? What do you mean, you're on an airplane?'

'I'm on the runway at Charles de Gaulle airport. I'm about to fly to Dubai.'

'No, no, Alexis. You need to come back. You're ill.'

'Well, obviously I'm not coming back. I'm going to Dubai. And I'll be staying overseas until you remove the section.'

'Don't threaten us.'

'I not threatening you,' I said. 'It's a fact. Remove the section.' The nurse asked me to come back a few more times.

The airplane taxied along the runway. I felt something like excitement or maybe happiness build. I was pressed into my seat as the airplane left the ground and reached altitude. I really cried.

After a long flight I landed in Dubai. I was quite anxious, but it was all good. The French police had said that if I landed anywhere in Europe, the flag on my passport would show. But landing out of Europe would be fine.

I asked them, 'Are you sure? Because I'm landing in Dubai, and I'll bet the residents of Dubai don't have a soft spot for escaped psychiatric patients.'

They said, 'No, honestly, it will be fine.'

'Are you sure? I could connect in Ethiopia if I wanted.'

'No, it will be fine.'

And it was fine. I walked straight through the Dubai immigration. No flag appeared. I got on the plane for Africa.

As we neared Lagos and began our descent, I filled out the landing card. I was worried again. The card asked, 'Have you committed a crime, or do you have a mental illness?'

I wrote no. I don't have a mental illness and I haven't committed a crime. I thought back to the incidents with Judy and Georgia and felt a little cross. I put these thoughts out of my head.

While I stood waiting to disembark I asked the air hostess, 'What's the immigration like here?' Naturally, I was scared again.

She said, 'I don't really know, because as cabin crew we pretty much just walk through it.'

This lovely Nigerian guy next to me said, 'You know, you just have to relax. It's Africa.'

At first, I thought it was an odd response to a question about immigration. However, he was right, and his statement has stuck with me. I thought, *Yeah. That's what I will do. I'm going to relax because I'm in Lagos. I'm in fucking Lagos!*

He said, 'This is a relaxed country.'

And it is.

I got off the plane. The heat of the African sun hit me. I looked up and the sky was big, not a cloud to be seen. I walked the short distance along the arrivals section, passing tourists bound for the West, no doubt. The terminal was basic; little lighting, no music, no TVs. It was just a building.

Arriving at immigration I was greeted with a familiar scene of complete chaos. I was reminded of my days in Asia and felt at home.

Passengers were pushing one another to get to the row of desks. There was no yellow line like in France. Instead it was whomever made eye contact with the official got to go first.

When I had pushed my way to the front I gave the official my immigration card and passport. He gave my passport a cursory glance before asking me for the $50 for my visa. He took my passport and gestured for me to join a crowd of people waiting for their passports back.

I waited for about an hour. Every 10 minutes, an immigration officer would come out of his booth and shout a list of names handing out the respective passports. Eventually, I got mine.

I exited the airport and Jaz was standing there with her driver, waving at me like crazy. It was hot, and I was glad to get into her air-conditioned Land Rover.

The journey was interesting, to say the least. For an hour, we weaved in and out of traffic, with people trying to sell us things on the road. Finally, we travelled along a dirt track riddled with potholes to Jaz's compound. We entered the large gates operated by a security team and pulled up to her house.

The driver got out of the car and took my luggage. Jaz's house is a four-bedroom, semi-detached with a large garden and shared swimming pool. Dickie, her husband, was not yet home, and I took the time to explain to Jaz a little bit about why I was there. She was shocked.

Later that evening, I Skyped with my family. My mum was still crying. Dad was relieved I had made it. The rehab unit had been in contact with him. When asked by the nurse what he was going to do about my escape, he told her, 'I am very pleased. I shall probably have a nice glass of wine and sleep well tonight.' I read this in my clinical notes.

I also Skyped with Jenny. They had enjoyed being in France and had visited some World War One sites they hadn't seen in a while. When they got home Jenny and David spoke to their lawyer. They were likely to be liable for prosecution for six months. If I had run away and committed suicide, I reckon they would have been prosecuted. If it went horribly wrong and I came back and was ill, they might be prosecuted. Thankfully, my life just got better and better. They deserve a medal for what they did.

CHAPTER 62

At Jaz's

When I landed at Jaz's, it was like I was transported in a time machine back to my days working alongside her as my colleague. In Asia, Jaz and I taught in the same school. Often after a long day in the classroom, we would meet up at her house or mine and watch dramas like *Grey's Anatomy* or *24*.

Jaz was non-judgemental and didn't play 20 questions with me. She let me tell her why I was in Lagos in my own time. She's not the pushy type and doesn't relish drama. Instead, she is outgoing and friendly, even to those she doesn't know. Jaz will meet somebody on a plane and say, 'Oh, come and stay with us.' Dickie never quite likes it when she does that.

Dickie is a level-headed, intelligent, gentle man. He works in exporting crude oil around the world. Where they live, oil is a main export.

Monday to Friday, Dickie would work from six o'clock in the morning until three o'clock the following morning. He left early to avoid traffic. I would be up watching TV and would say goodbye before he left. Jaz loves her bed and would sleep in until about ten o'clock every morning. Because they had just moved to Lagos, she hadn't yet found work. It was nice to have her company.

Jaz introduced me to her new friends. There were different expat groups every day. They varied from "ladies who lunch" to a book group. There was even a mosaic group. Although this life sounds privileged, which of course it was, it's not that easy to be an expat wife in Africa. It was lonely sometimes, especially for a newbie. Jaz was still establishing herself in the local community. So, it was ideal I was doing this alongside her. I had to concoct a story about why I was in Africa. Initially I told people I was visiting. After a month, I told them I was looking for work.

I felt like I had landed in an oasis, especially when I strolled along the white sand beach in 30-degree heat. The beach was a five-minute walk from the house. The air was clean. The roads were dirt tracks, with potholes in the red soil. One thing I love so much about Nigeria is the big skies, blue and cloudless.

The neighbourhood where Jaz lived was quiet and safe. In the compound I swam every day in the open-air pool and then went to the gym.

There were very few shops around. But there was a European supermarket a short walk from Jaz's house. There I bought basic foodstuffs easily without feeling overstimulated. It was very autism friendly. On the walk home, I would greet monkeys playing in the trees.

During the first 24 hours of my time there, I told Dickie and Jaz the very basics of what had happened.

Dickie said, 'Lex, you seem to be the same person I knew four years ago.'

I could tell they were worried about my presence, so I told them, 'You haven't broken the law by having me here because you're not in England, and you haven't helped me escape. If this goes wrong, and it's not fine, then I'll leave. And if at any time you want me to leave, then I will.' We kind of agreed on that informally.

Jaz said, 'No, no. Lexi, you can stay as long as you need to.'

'That's really kind, but I just plan on staying a month or so.' I told them I knew I would go through withdrawals because I had been on such a huge amount of drugs and David had been clear about this before I left.

I'd already done my research and found that there is not much psychiatry in Nigeria. This meant there was no chance of tapering off the drugs. I was going to go "cold turkey".

In the house was Jessie, the dog, with her unconditional positive regard for any human, no matter their mental health status. And two cats called Bugger and Sweetie. Jaz had found these animals on the side of the road one day in Asia. She couldn't resist bringing home strays. The cat Bugger was a true bugger. He was vicious and unpredictable. However, I loved him.

Bugger had half a tail and looks like a street tomcat. He was almost dead when Jaz rescued him. She took him in to Dickie, who was in bed. Jaz put Bugger beside him, this mangy, injured kitten full of fleas.

Dickie said, 'What are you doing? Get him off the bed. He's got fleas.'

'Oh, but Dickie, he is dying.'

Dickie said, 'Oh, Jaz,' and resigned himself – they spent almost $1,000 on the cat. Now, whenever Dickie sees Jaz eyeing up a cat, he starts saying, 'No, no.'

The dog Jessie and these cats have more air miles than most people. They've lived in three continents and are privileged street animals. I made friends with the dog immediately. She didn't care what I was doing.

During my incarceration, I had been under tremendous pressure to act a certain way, to talk a certain way. Now if I overslept in the morning because I'd been awake all night, no one said, 'Oh, you're up half an hour late. What's wrong? What's wrong?' Or, 'You've had two cups of hot chocolate before bed. You're only supposed to have one.' Or, 'Why are you going to bed at 10 o'clock, Alexis?' Or, 'Why have you been up three times tonight?' Nobody cared. No one took notes. Nobody would pop around to see me or phone me or threaten me.

I realised that it wasn't weird to wake up 45 minutes late on a Tuesday. There was nothing wrong with that. If I ran for 30 minutes because I couldn't be bothered to run for 40, no one was asking, 'Why are you back early?' Interrogation had been non-stop before. But now it was non-existent. I could just live my life.

CHAPTER 63

Cold Turkey

The first 48 hours were fine. I was tired and mentally exhausted from what I had just done, but otherwise I was in good health. Then the withdrawals started.

I had been on many drugs over the three-and-a-half years I was incarcerated. I saw from research that the hardest to come off were benzodiazepines and SSRIs. I had no choice but to stop everything. I left the UK with no supply and in Lagos there are no psychiatric drugs. My approach to withdrawal was resolute. I knew that I had to make it or succumb to a life incarcerated.

Given my new-found freedom, I was positive for the first time in years. I started the withdrawal as a bit of a challenge – a challenge I felt good about. Insomnia and dizziness were just the start. While they weren't pleasant, they were bearable.

Then, just days later, my skin started fizzing. A hot, fiery feeling ran in my veins. My brain felt as if it was being zapped by electricity every few hours, sometimes as often as every few minutes. And this was only the start.

One of the most uncomfortable symptoms was a continual pressure in my ears. It felt like I was deep in a swimming pool. No matter how many times I tried to clear my ears, immediately it would come back with the horrendous pressure. I thought it was never going away. I phoned David and he said to monitor it and keep records of what was happening, which I never did – don't tell him. That was the last thing I wanted to do. He said it was important. I was like, uuuhhhh. I couldn't even bloody take a drink, let alone do anything else.

In a matter of days, I was curled up in a fetal position with sharp, piercing, insufferable pain everywhere. I was sweating constantly, and it wasn't from the heat of the sun. I had to change my clothes all the time. I hardly had any clothes, so Jaz lent me hers.

My body couldn't be still. Akathisia is a strong compulsion. The result of antipsychotic withdrawal, this urge to be in motion can never be satisfied. In my room at the bottom of Jaz's house, I swayed from foot to foot. In worse times, I paced while standing. When I needed to rest I lay down but lifted and lowered my legs as if I was walking. When I was sitting watching TV, I jigged my legs over the couch. The need to move never ended. It took no rest even during the night.

These changes from brain-altering substances didn't revert easily. The first few weeks were like years. I looked terrible and felt like death. One day, it became so unbearable that I called Oxlip. I'm not sure why – I don't know what I wanted or needed. But I was in excruciating pain. Although I was certain I wouldn't die, the physical pain felt like I was on my way. What they said, and what they didn't say, toughened my resolve.

'Come home,' they said. 'What you are doing is dangerous,' they said. 'You are susceptible to psychosis. You are ill and need help.'

Do I? Do I really need your help? What will you do? Put me back on the drugs? Lock me up?

I don't think I would ever have been drug free in England. If I had tried to come off the drugs there, I wouldn't have made it. There's no way they would've let me go through a four-week withdrawal. I had a choice. Go back or stay here.

I made a life-changing decision that day. I finally understood that to live means to suffer. Truly, I had never felt so bad. The pain was unrivalled. When I gave birth, when Josh died and during the difficult months that followed, I realised now I had never been pathologically ill. I learnt that day the important lesson of enduring suffering. I didn't like it! Who would? But I also knew I didn't need professional help. I had to stay in the moment and accept my situation. I thought back to the lessons in York about "radical acceptance" of my situation. Any resistance to what was happening or desire to change would bring more suffering, as the Psychologist Felicity would reason.

So, I endured. The sweating, the brain zaps, the fizzing skin, the pain in every muscle, insomnia, the unbearable need to move, headaches, the pressure in my ears, and everything else.

It felt so weird to get the dog and go out. It was nice not to be on my own, because I hadn't been free in that way for years. I didn't have to ask, and I could come back when I wanted. It was such a strange adjustment. I think if I had not been suffering the horrific withdrawals, it would've been a bigger adjustment. But I was just trying to concentrate on standing up straight, and not falling over when I had the brain zaps. Jessie was great company. I felt safe with her. When my skin would fizz up like I was a shaken bottle of Coke, she would be by my side offering support.

At one point I called David. 'I can't stand this. It's awful.'

He asked, 'Do you want to come home?'

I said, 'Hell, no. I do not want to come home.'

I looked up withdrawals on the internet. When you get an extreme reaction, it's called antidepressant discontinuation syndrome. But this wasn't just from an antidepressant. It was antipsychotics, Ritalin, amphetamines, zopiclone, antihistamines, and others. There were multiple reports it could actually last for years. There've been so many lawsuits against the drug companies related to SSRI withdrawals.

Nobody says it takes two or three weeks as drug companies claim, so I had to prepare for the worst.

David asked, 'Are you prepared, Lexi? You could fly down to South Africa and pick up some drugs and withdraw steadily.'

I said, 'No. I've read if you do that it just prolongs the agony.' It was agony, and extremely frightening. When I stood up to go out, I couldn't move because I was in so much pain. I would get up in the night. I couldn't just stay in my room, so I would sit and have a chat with Jessie. Pet therapy was way better than with most psychologists anyway.

A few weeks later, on a day in hell, I suddenly realised that I hadn't been in pain for about 10 minutes. It was a staggering insight that brought feelings of disbelief. Although I wasn't used to the pain, I was living with it.

This was the first of increasingly frequent windows of reprieve. The duration and frequency of brain zaps became more bearable. I went longer without being so dizzy I would stumble. I read that you get bigger windows. You might get a window of an hour where you have no symptoms. My windows were getting longer – two hours, then three hours. One day I noticed that I hadn't had a brain zap. As soon as the windows were big enough, reaching up to 12 hours before I'd get a zap, my mind was clear. The clouds were gone, and I could think. These gaps allowed me time to leave my room to get a drink. Then I could go outside and enjoy the blue sky and the sun. Finally, I could walk to the local shop. My appetite increased. And I slept one night in every three instead of one in every five or seven.

I thought my withdrawals were extreme. I now know from blogs and forums that they were normal. There is a lot of support and reassurance on the web from people who have suffered terrible withdrawals. Unfortunately, long-term withdrawal effects of SSRIs are not recognised by organised psychiatry. Withdrawal is a lonely place. It is helpful, when you already feel like an alien, to realise you are not alone. You are not weird; it isn't you that is faulty. It's that drug companies and organised psychiatry are hiding this aspect of people's experience.

I hadn't felt so positive for years. I regained a sense of safety in the world. When I left the UK, I had instantly gotten so much back. My freedom meant everything was possible again. I could nurture a tender sprout of passion for life and hope for the future. I might once again be a mother, a daughter, a friend. I might even one day use my voice to help others suffering as I had suffered.

AFTERWORD

It's been more than two years since I escaped from Oxlip. I have a highly skilled job working for a global education giant. The salary is good, which is useful since my ADLs are still substandard, so I can afford household help and a nanny to help with my daughter.

But even though things are good, it is hard to ignore the fact that no one representing the mental health system has taken responsibility for the acts inflicted on me, or taken any measures to prevent further harm. In fact, they had planned to start all over again if or when I returned to England.

I spent 115 days from 17th May 2016 begging for my right to challenge my Section 3. This meant I was forced to stay overseas. Luckily, I had the financial resources and mental fortitude to remain out of the country.

In full knowledge of the progress I made in securing full time professional employment, running my own house, and single-handedly parenting my four-year-old child, the NHS plan was to detain me on arrival and assess me in a psychiatric intensive care unit.

So, I attended a hearing tribunal via Skype.

The written evidence submitted by Dr Malvada was as follows:

I can only make a recommendation for Alexis remaining on section based on the nature of her mental disorder. Since the end of 2012, following the death of her brother Joshua, Alexis has been in hospital nearly all of the time. On occasions, she has been discharged to the community but readmitted soon after as she was not coping and her behaviours was putting her and others at risk. Also, the risk of suicide and to the safety of others has remained high.

All she had to say was, 'Yes, she'll be going to Ivy Suite.'

My solicitor asked, 'And the panel will not think that's a slight escalation to send her to a secure ward?'

The panel could only respond, 'Uh, yes, perhaps it is.'

There was no clear therapeutic purpose to my treatment but to try to eliminate autism. Now my brain is clear of drugs and I've had time to think. I am now much stronger. I want to advocate for my right to exist without fear that because of my uniqueness people might terrorise me, permanently altering my mind in the most intrusive and irreversible ways. At present, this right still does not exist for me or others like me. My story is common. What happened to me was not my personal failure and understanding this has helped me to heal.

Trauma is the most profound harm caused. I have developed stress reactions of daily flashbacks, phobia of uniformed staff, police cars and sirens, and avoidance of conditions that remind me of my time in wards.

I know if I get cold while asleep this can trigger a flashback of my stay in that freezing seclusion room. I am very anxious when I return to the UK. The experience of being locked inside a cage has had a severe psychological impact on me.

I wanted to believe the system heals, but the fact is, it's an unnatural invasion that penetrates every encounter, thought, feeling. You have little control over anything.

It was a shock to come from a fairly safe, comfortable, and autonomous life to one characterised by subversion and control. Filled with anxiety, I was afraid of the system and what was happening. In so many ways, psychiatry created my problems.

The chaotic ordeal created a potent culture of submission to the mental health system and to other more powerful patients. Shredding of personal autonomy facilitates this. Relationships between staff and patients are contrived and inauthentic, since the entire system is designed to denigrate. The very essence of who you are is taken away.

Once free, it only took a few months to find myself again. I don't know how to explain this. Although I am changed forever, it's hard to describe such a dramatic alteration in personality. I think I must have subconsciously slipped into the role of lesser human, mentally-ill defective person to save myself from existential crisis. By accepting this diminished status, I was more able to resurrect my self-worth when I was no longer oppressed.

Sadly, there are also significant social challenges from being involved with the mental health system. In many professions like mine, you must do a medical. In the UK, this always includes a medical history. Every occupational health form I have filled in has asked whether I have been diagnosed with a mental illness, as well as whether or not I've ever self-harmed. The Section 136s, when I was held by police, might show up on police checks. The "assault" on Judy in which I was the "alleged perpetrator" will show up on my DBS Police check. Needless to say, this affects my employability. The stress of thinking about these things compounds the trauma and embeds it deeper. And in my new life outside the UK, I hide my mental health history completely because I am afraid for my job.

Then there are challenges associated with my diminished self in the family home and community. Once a respected member of both, I am now the crazy person people murmur about as I pass. The damage to my relationships are in some instances irreparable.

*

Today, I am glad I did not die. I tell people in situations similar to mine to try to find meaning in the degradation and purpose in those shameful units. Without the suffering, I would never have known the depths of my indomitable spirit.

Not a day goes by in which I don't think about what happened. I am astonished that society has been duped by a system so discriminatory and fallacious. Yet, more recently, I have hope that things are changing for the better. More attention is being given to mental health. It is becoming harder for people to dismiss stories such as mine as tendentious and atypical in a system which is otherwise very compassionate. In refusing to do, so we can begin to be reflective, challenge the status quo and improve lives.

I was pleased to read in 2018 of two landmark reports containing data indicating that UK mental health hospitals were falling far below acceptable standards of care and human rights. The first report was independently commissioned by Theresa May (The Independent Review of the Mental Health Act)[5] and the second by the World Health Organisation (Mental health care institutions in Europe well below standard – new WHO *assessment*)[6].

Both reports confirm my experience; that there are serious problems with the Mental Health Act. Dr Sri Kalidindi, a spokeswoman for the Royal College of Psychiatrists in the UK who wasn't involved in the WHO study said that the inequality was clear and treatment of persons who are most vulnerable was unacceptable (CNN report, 6th June 2018)[7].

Among the more severe transgressions documented in both reports were that people were subject to distressing experiences, for example: witnessing physical violence, verbal abuse, and threatening behaviour. Use of restraints to manage difficult behaviour, coercive reward and punishment systems for access to open-air leave or family contact, bullying, and harassment were found to be far too common. There is also the sexual abuse of female patients, restrictions on communication, and little access to meaningful daily activities. All of this has been shown to lead to physical and psychological harm. All of this was clearly documented in the reports.

The government's Interim report findings show that while the Mental Health Act can save lives, many under it felt mistreated, with two-thirds expressing strong views saying they were not treated with dignity and that their human rights were not respected.

CHANGE – A WAY FORWARDS

We must ask: Can society do better than this current system?

Psychiatric services are dilapidated. It's surprisingly hard to get access to the skeletal system unless you have the resources to pay privately or you are considered a danger. Even if you are deemed "dangerous", treatment is hard to come by and you are more likely to be given drugs and told to "get on with it".

Having witnessed my own loving, supportive, privileged family fall apart over my emotional distress and substandard care in institutions, I have wondered whether there is hope for this broken system.

I have listened to people who wish to do away with psychiatry. I have considered their arguments and asked myself – If I could go back and receive the care I needed, with genuine understanding and a robust support package, would I? Of course I would! And so., when there is nothing else to replace psychiatry, I don't think it wise to go about trying to destroy it.

THE STARTING POINT FOR CHANGE: EXPANDING THE SINGLE STORY

When I started work in Lagos I had a week of induction training. During this week, we heard a lecture on single stories from the Nigerian novelist Chimamanda Ngozi Adichie via a TED talk.

Adichie discussed what she calls the "danger of a single story". I was enamoured as she described how subtle power structures are capable of creating one dangerously simplified perspective of a person or culture. She says if 'You show a people as one thing, as only one thing, over and over again ... that is what they become.'[8]

That sounds familiar.

The systemic injustice I experienced was to a great extent caused by the biological explanation for mental disorder. Those experiencing extreme states of being, those with issues or differences in thinking or behaviour, are seen to be faulty. The faultiness is understood as neurons firing too much or not enough, chemical imbalances or something of the sort. Medication is often thought to be needed for life. The "mental patients" are dangerous, a risk, not capable of leading a normal life, a drain on society.

THE DANGER OF THE SINGLE STORY

I know for some people getting a diagnosis can be reassuring. Most people that take psychiatric medication believe it is designed for their "illness" or "disorder". They are led to believe if they follow the treatment plan they will get well. This concept is appealing. It is simple. It also provides a reason for the dysregulation. It means that the problem is no more their fault than if they had a broken leg. And yes, it can have benefits like getting people the financial support and resources and treatment they may need.

For me, it isn't a case of which theory I most like. It's rather, what is the truth, and what are the effects of truth / mistruth?

Mental illnesses are a matter of opinion. That is why I had, for over two years, a different diagnosis from almost every doctor I saw.

Yet even in the early days, the idea of reducing myself to a diagnosis never sat well with me. It was always too simplistic and didn't take account of much of what was going on in my life. I remembered only when I escaped the system that I was a well-educated, professional lady, a sister, a daughter, a mother,

315

and friend. All of these roles defined me and fleshed out my life far more accurately than a collection of symptoms assigned to an arbitrary label. And yet it is this label that is so powerful and comes to define you inside the system.

Unfortunately, I was powerless to counter the medical narratives and correct the biological commentary – to realise that my story and subjective experience had little to do with the current disorder I happened to be labelled with. It was Dr Liz Hadley in York that encouraged me to talk and allowed me to explain my attributional model. She recognised my experiential knowledge. Dr Hadley is an example of someone who appreciated human diversity and showed compassion to those in need of it. This is a good starting point for improvement as it expands the single story.

A WAY FORWARDS – EXPANDING PSYCHIATRY'S SINGLE STORY

People need to know that the medical model isn't all it's cracked up to be. Diagnosis, however helpful or unhelpful, should not be presented as facts. Drugs should not be the treatment of choice. The truth of these two powerhouses should be told to patients that receive psychiatric help. Genuine informed consent must be attained before drugs aredished out.

We need to embrace the psychosocial model. The totality of a person, their pain and suffering, and their lived environment cannot be understood by only considering the single story. We must take account of context. We must care about the details and open our hearts and minds to the person's life if we really want to help.

Let's look at ourselves in a compassionate and empathic way and stop reducing ourselves to a label. We are so much more. The publication of the Power Threat Meaning Framework (PTMF) in 2018 creates a new and more hopeful narrative. It is based on four key questions[9]:

- What has happened to you? (How is power operating in your life?)

- How did it affect you? (What kind of threats does this pose?)

- What sense did you make of It? (What is the meaning of these situations and experiences to you?)

- What did you have to do to survive? (What kinds of threat response are you using?)

Dr Lucy Johnstone, Consultant Clinical Psychologist and others who were instrumental in creating this framework said:

> *The Power Threat Meaning Framework can be used as a way of helping people to create more hopeful narratives or stories about their lives and the difficulties they have faced or are still facing, instead of seeing themselves as blameworthy, weak, deficient or "mentally ill". (BPS, 2018)*

The PTMF is supportive of people's struggles and could be the springboard for transformation in the way we approach psychological distress. One in four people are suffering. It's likely we all know somebody in real pain. Society has a responsibility to embrace this paradigm shift and look beyond the dominant single story. This is not going to be easy. Exploring the impact of trauma, abuse, or ordinary stresses on experience and behaviour requires fortitude and bravery. But it seems to me the human thing to do.

*

Psychiatry, with its labels, drugs, and stigma, needs to be the last line of defence for the vast majority. The truth of psychiatry's single story, so well disguised, needs to be made common knowledge and genuine informed consent to treatment an option. The paradigm shift offered by the PTMF should be embraced as a method of expanding the single story. If and when this happens, so will psychiatry's capacity to truly help.

If you found this book interesting ...
why not read these next?

Teacup In A Storm

Finding My Psychiatrist

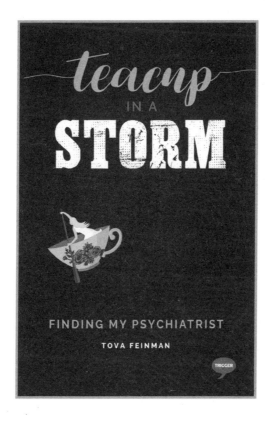

Wracked with trauma from childhood abuse, Tova sought therapy to soothe her mind. However, it is not as easy as simply finding a person to talk to ...

Sex, Suicide & Serotonin

Taking Myself Apart,
Putting Myself Back Together

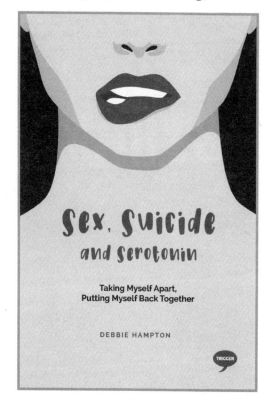

When Debbie Hampton took the mix of wine and drugs that nearly killed her, she didn't ever want to wake up – but she did, and her problems were only just beginning. In this book, Debbie tells the inspirational story of how she forged a new life for herself.

Walk A Mile Book

Tales of a Wandering Loon

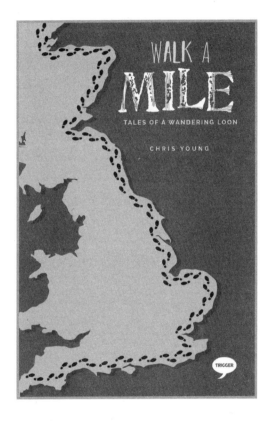

Chris Young was all too aware of the stigma surrounding BPD. And so he decided to walk around the edge of the UK – as many with mental illness feel they belong on the edge of society – and challenge mental health stigma, one conversation at a time.

REFERENCES

1 Health and Social Care Information Centre (2015). Learning Disability Census 2015: almost half of inpatients with learning disabilities common to each census since 2013. Retrieved from http://content.digital.nhs.uk/article/6874/Learning-Disability-Census-2015-almost-half-of-inpatients-with-learning-disabilities-common-to-each-census-since-2013. Accessed 5th July 2017.

2 **Miserandino, C.** (2003). "The Spoon Theory". Retrieved from https://butyoudontlooksick.com/articles/written-by-christine/the-spoon-theory/. Accessed 5th July 2017.

3 **Lipsky, D and Richards, W.S.** (2009). *Managing Meltdowns: Using the S.C.A.R.E.D Calming Technique with Children and Adults with Autism.* Jessica Kingsley Publishers.

4 **Mental Health Act 1983, s.128.**

5 **UK Government (2018).** The Independent Review of the Mental Health Act (England & Wales). Retrieved from https://assets.publishing.service.gov.uk/government/uploads/system/uploads/attachment_data/file/703919/The_independent_Mental_Health_Act_review__interim_report_01_05_2018.pdf. Accessed 7th June 2018.

6 **World Health Organisation Regional Office for Europe** (2018). Mental health, human rights and standards of care:

assessment of the quality of institutional care for adults with psychosocial and intellectual disabilities in the WHO European Region. Retrieved from www.euro.who.int/__data/ assets/pdf_file/0017/373202/mental-health-programme-eng. pdf?ua=1 Accessed 13th May 2018.

7 **Smith, R.** (2018). European mental health institutions fall "far below the standard", WHO reports. Retrieved from https://edition.cnn.com/2018/06/06/health/who-mental-health-institutions-intl/index.html Accessed 13th May 2018.

8 **Adichie, CN.** (2009). The danger of a single story. [Online video]. Available at: www.ted.com/talks/chimamanda_adichie_the_danger_of_a_single_story Accessed 10th April 2018.

9 **British Psychological Association** (2018). Introducing the Power Threat Meaning Framework. Retrieved from www.bps.org.uk/news-and-policy/introducing-power-threat-meaning-framework. Accessed 23rd March 2018.

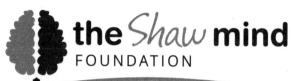

the *Shaw* mind
FOUNDATION

Creating hope for children,
adults and families

Sign up to our charity, The Shaw Mind Foundation
www.shawmindfoundation.org
and keep in touch with us; we would love to hear
from you.

*We aim to bring to an end the suffering and despair caused
by mental health issues. Our goal is to make help and support
available for every single person in society, from all walks of
life. We will never stop offering hope. These are our promises.*

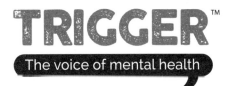

www.triggerpublishing.com

Trigger is a publishing house devoted to opening conversations about mental health. We tell the stories of people who have suffered from mental illnesses and recovered, so that others may learn from them.

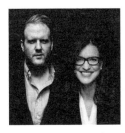

Adam Shaw is a worldwide mental health advocate and philanthropist. Now in recovery from mental health issues, he is committed to helping others suffering from debilitating mental health issues through the global charity he co-founded, The Shaw Mind Foundation. www.shawmindfoundation.org

Lauren Callaghan (CPsychol, PGDipClinPsych, PgCert, MA (hons), LLB (hons), BA), born and educated in New Zealand, is an innovative industry-leading psychologist based in London, United Kingdom. Lauren has worked with children and young people, and their families, in a number of clinical settings providing evidence based treatments for a range of illnesses, including anxiety and obsessional problems. She was a psychologist at the specialist national treatment centres for severe obsessional problems in the UK and is renowned as an expert in the field of mental health, recognised for diagnosing and successfully treating OCD and anxiety related illnesses in particular. In addition to appearing as a treating clinician in the critically acclaimed and BAFTA award-winning documentary *Bedlam*, Lauren is a frequent guest speaker on mental health conditions in the media and at academic conferences. Lauren also acts as a guest lecturer and honorary researcher at the Institute of Psychiatry Kings College, UCL.

Please visit the link below:

www.triggerpublishing.com

Join us and follow us...

@triggerpub

Search for us on Facebook